T0144849

BASIC HEALTH PUBLICATIONS USER'S GUIDE

TO CARNOSINE

Learn How This Super-Nutrient Can Fight Aging, Boost Your Immunity, and Prevent Disease.

MARIE MONEYSMITH
JACK CHALLEM Series Editor

The information contained in this book is based upon the research and personal and professional experiences of the author. It is not intended as a substitute for consulting with your physician or other healthcare provider. Any attempt to diagnose and treat an illness should be done under the direction of a healthcare professional.

The publisher does not advocate the use of any particular healthcare protocol but believes the information in this book should be available to the public. The publisher and author are not responsible for any adverse effects or consequences resulting from the use of the suggestions, preparations, or procedures discussed in this book. Should the reader have any questions concerning the appropriateness of any procedures or preparations mentioned, the author and the publisher strongly suggest consulting a professional healthcare advisor.

Series Editor: Jack Challem
Editor: Susan Andrews
Typesetter: Gary A. Rosenberg
Series Cover Designer: Mike Stromberg

Basic Health Publications User's Guides are published by Basic Health Publications, Inc.

CONTENTS

INTRODUCTION

Carnosine may be one of the best-kept secrets in the supplement world. In fact, it has such a low profile that when people first hear its name, they often confuse it with *carnitine,* which is a very different substance.

Technically, carnosine is not a vitamin or mineral. It is a is dipeptide, but don't be put off by the unfamiliar terminology. A dipeptide is simply a compound created by the union of two amino acids, in this case, alanine and histidine.

Amino acids are best known as the building blocks of protein. But in the case of carnosine, the pairing creates a compound substance with a special synergy that takes it far beyond protein creation. Carnosine has shown great promise for improving all-around health, slowing the aging process, and even treating such difficult conditions as Alzheimer's disease, Parkinson's disease, and autism.

Why is a supplement as powerful as carnosine not better known? Even though there are more than 1,000 studies focusing on carnosine, most of them were done abroad, primarily in Russia, and more recently in Europe and other parts of Asia. As a result, American medical experts and the media have largely been unaware of the extensive research on this potent substance. That is likely to change in the near future, however. Carnosine simply has too much to offer to a wide range of the population to remain in the background.

Take, for example, the baby-boom generation, composed of millions of men and women born between 1946 and 1964. The baby boomers are taking the clichés about growing old and turning them upside down. Thanks to advances in anti-aging medicine, not to mention plastic surgery, the baby boomers are not going to go quietly into old age. In fact, they seem to be determined to actively engage in hand-to-hand combat with Father Time and Mother Nature, with no plans to surrender any time soon.

Not surprisingly, anti-aging medicine is the fastest-growing segment of preventive health care in this century, a multibillion-dollar business fueled in large part by the baby boomers' reluctance to grow old. For some people, anti-aging is not a matter of quantity but quality. They're more interested in how well they live, rather than how long, so staying healthy and robust is the primary goal. For others, maintaining youth means avoiding wrinkles and gray hair, as well as creaky joints and "senior moments."

Where does carnosine fit into this picture? Everywhere. Let's start with heart disease, the nation's number-one killer. Carnosine enhances heart health in several ways, including interference with the production of LDL (low-density lipoprotein, or "bad") cholesterol. It helps keep blood vessels supple and "young," as well.

Aside from heart disease, carnosine helps us maintain good health in other ways. For example, carnosine has special antioxidant abilities that enable it to protect our cells and their contents, including our genes, from damaging rogue molecules known as free radicals. Although assaults by free radicals affect us on a microscopic level and aren't immediately apparent, illness will eventually result. Cancer, for example, is a disease that by and large takes years to develop. During that time, the body's cells are quietly being altered by compounds that could be eliminated by substances such as carnosine. In fact, many experts say carnosine could become a potent weapon in the war against cancer.

Carnosine also has an important function with regard to aging. According to one theory of aging, free-radical damage is linked to many of the devastating diseases associated with advancing years. All antioxidants play a major role in good health at any age, but become increasingly important as the years pass. Vitamins A, C, and E and the minerals selenium and zinc are well-known antioxidants. A powerhouse antioxidant, carnosine supports the work of these and other free-radical fighters.

However, carnosine goes a step further, by preventing a serious form of protein damage known as glycation. Free radicals and antioxidants have become household words, but many people are unaware of the harmful effects of glycation, an irregular bonding of sugar and protein with extensive health consequences, including hastening the aging process. Recognizing how glycation occurs and how it can be prevented—or at least minimized—with carnosine can help avoid the damage that accrues with time.

But carnosine's antiglycation benefits don't end there. People with insulin resistance, a major factor in a condition known as Syndrome X, and those with diabetes are also prone to glycation. In their cases, glycation stimulates the aging process, but fortunately, they can gain protection from carnosine.

Carnosine provides other anti-aging benefits.

For instance, although scientists are not sure exactly how it works yet, carnosine has been shown to rejuvenate old cells and also help them live longer, an ability that could help keep the body in peak shape in later years. Carnosine also interferes with the creation of beta-amyloid, a substance associated with Alzheimer's disease, and carnosine eyedrops fight the formation of cataracts, the leading cause of vision difficulties in the elderly. Additionally, as a cream, carnosine can be applied to the skin to minimize wrinkles and age spots.

Although osteoporosis is now a household word, the Centers for Disease Control (CDC) recently named a condition known as "sarcopenia" as one of the top five health risks among older adults. Sarcopenia is a combination of the gradual erosion of lean muscle and the accumulation of fat that eventually causes frailty in older people, and is believed to contribute to bone-breaking falls. After age forty, the typical adult loses from one-fourth to one-third of a pound of muscle each year and gains about the same amount in body fat. The result: overall weakness that can be immobilizing. Stairs become a challenge. Even getting up from a chair may require assistance. Strength training is the best-known way to counteract sarcopenia, and carnosine can be a valuable ally. Studies have shown that carnosine can rejuvenate and strengthen muscles, as well as increase energy and endurance, among athletes and nonathletes alike. For a generation of aging baby boomers, carnosine may help them avoid falling victim to one of the most common indignities suffered by the elderly—loss of independence.

Similarly, inflammation has recently been acknowledged to be closely linked to a wide range of serious, chronic health conditions and diseases. Here again, carnosine can help minimize inflammation through its role as an antioxidant and by removing some of the substances responsible for inflammation.

Carnosine plays other roles in good health. For example, it has been shown to help wounds heal faster, both on the skin's surface and internally, in the form of ulcers. Carnosine is found in high concentrations in muscle tissue, and, not surprisingly, it has been used for years by athletes and bodybuilders to overcome muscle fatigue. While it is considered a worthwhile addition to any athlete's regimen, it can also help the average person work out more efficiently, a factor that can contribute to weight loss. And in our country, with more than 60 percent of the adult population overweight or obese, that is no small advantage.

Although research is in its early stages, several studies show that neurodegenerative ailments, such as Parkinson's disease, respond well to carnosine. And a recent clinical trial in Chicago found that carnosine improves symptoms of autism in children, creating tremendous excitement for the growing number of families challenged by this condition.

Store shelves are filled with supplements making claims backed by only a handful of studies. By contrast, there is no shortage of carnosine research. In literally hundreds of studies, minor side effects have been found only rarely, and even then only at very high doses. Carnosine also has no known drug interactions. In fact, if carnosine has a downside, researchers have yet to find it.

Make no mistake—carnosine is not a miraculous wonder drug that can add years to your life or make up for a bad diet, sedentary lifestyle, or other irresponsible behavior. But it is shaping up as an essential ingredient in good health, with an important role in keeping us fit and feeling our best.

CHAPTER 1

ALL ABOUT CARNOSINE

Just prior to the discovery of vitamins—in 1900, to be exact—carnosine was isolated from muscle tissue by Russian researchers. Although carnosine has been the subject of hundreds of studies since then, most of them were conducted in Russia. Political tensions between the United States and the former Soviet Union prevented the exchange of this sort of information. It was not until quite recently that scientists worldwide learned about carnosine. Since then, it has developed a small but growing reputation as a substance that improves cardiovascular health, strengthens the immune system, encourages healing of skin wounds and ulcers, and fights a wide range of conditions associated with aging, from cellular deterioration to cataracts and wrinkles.

Carnosine is a small but versatile molecule. It is sometimes also referred to as beta-alanyl. In chemical terms, carnosine is actually made up of two different amino acids, alanine and histidine. Technically, this makes it a dipeptide, which simply means a combination of two amino acids. Carnosine-synthetase is the enzyme that helps join the two. At the other end of the spectrum, an enzyme known as carnosinase dissolves the union, leaving behind the two original amino acids.

Amino Acids
Most commonly known as the "building blocks" of proteins, but they have many other functions.

Where Carnosine Comes From

Muscle tissue is the primary source of carnosine, but not all muscle contains the same amount of the substance. Turkey, white-meat chicken, and beef from cattle's legs are rich in carnosine, as are a few types of fish, including sturgeon. Human skeletal muscle also contains carnosine, and levels are highest in muscles that contract, such as the biceps in the arms and calf muscles in the legs.

Carnosine is also heavily concentrated in the heart (which is a muscle), in the brain, and in cells that typically have long life spans, such as neurons. Like so many other beneficial substances, levels of carnosine in the body diminish as we age. Not surprisingly, low levels of carnosine in the lens of the eye have been found in cataract patients. At the same time, carnosine supplements have been found to prevent cataracts in animal studies, and a form of carnosine in eyedrops has shown promise for the treatment and prevention of cataracts.

Neuron
A nerve cell that sends and receives electrical signals throughout the body.

Understanding Amino Acids

To better understand carnosine and how it works in the body, we need to know a little about amino acids in general and carnosine's individual components in particular. Amino acids are most famous for being the "building blocks" of proteins found throughout our bodies. But this is only part of the story. While some amino acids help in protein production, others support the work of specific vitamins and minerals, serve as neurotransmitters (the chemical messengers that relay messages between nerve and brains cells), or play a role in metabolism.

Almost all the amino acids we need—roughly 80 percent—are produced in the liver when our bodies break down the protein we eat. The resulting amino acids are then recycled into other forms of protein that can be used to rebuild muscle, help bones grow, and maintain many normal bodily functions. The amino acids that cannot be manufactured in our bodies must come from food; these are known as essential amino acids.

Although diet is a major factor, levels of amino acid are also affected by other things, such as stress, aging, various prescription drugs, and poor digestion. These factors can also cause an imbalance among amino acids that could lead to health problems.

While eating a high-protein diet may seem like it would help avoid a shortage of amino acids, such a diet can overload the liver and kidneys. According to many experts, 50 grams of protein daily is sufficient, although many high-protein diets recommend more. (The body can only absorb 35 grams of protein at one meal.) A varied diet that provides correct proportions of carbohydrates, protein, and fats is much healthier indeed.

The Components of Carnosine

As you now know, carnosine is not a true amino acid, but a combination of alanine and histidine. Both of these substances have impressive abilities of their own. Being familiar with the components of carnosine will help you understand why this nutrient can accomplish so much in the body and why it is so highly regarded among researchers who have studied it.

All about Alanine

Alanine plays a whole host of vital roles in the

body. A nonessential amino acid first discovered in the late 1800s, alanine is used extensively throughout the body to build protein.

Another one of alanine's most significant functions occurs when we exercise. Vigorous activity demands the release of energy from protein in the muscles, a process that creates free radicals, dangerous toxins that can harm our cells. Alanine prevents the accumulation of these toxic substances. In addition, alanine aids in the metabolism of glucose and is used in supplement form by some diabetics to avoid low blood sugar (hypoglycemia).

Alanine is also involved in metabolizing tryptophan, an essential amino acid that helps produce serotonin, an important neurotransmitter that affects mood and sleep patterns.

The same form of alanine (beta-alanine) that is found in carnosine is also found in pantothenic acid, better known as vitamin B_5, a potent stress-fighting nutrient that is involved in development of hormones in the adrenal glands.

Hormones
Chemical messengers produced in the glands that travel through the bloodstream, delivering their messages.

Because prostate fluid contains alanine, some experts believe that a sufficient level of this amino acid is important for a properly functioning prostate. One study found that men with benign prostatic hyperplasia experienced symptom relief with supplements of alanine, glutamic acid, and glycine, two other amino acids.

Although alanine is clearly essential for good health, balance is important. Too much alanine, combined with low levels of the amino acids phenylalanine and tyrosine, has been found in people who have chronic fatigue syndrome or Epstein-Barr virus. Foods rich in alanine include meat, fish, chicken, dairy products, eggs, and avocados.

Help from Histidine

Unlike alanine, histidine is an essential amino acid, so we must obtain it from food or supplements. One of its primary roles is tissue growth and repair. Histidine has a special affinity for the myelin sheaths that safeguard our nerve cells. The creation of red and white blood cells, as well as certain digestive substances, requires histidine. In addition, this hardworking amino acid helps eliminate heavy metals from the body and helps reduce blood pressure.

Myelin
A layered fatty substance that covers and protects nerves.

Histidine can be converted to histamine, a compound produced by the immune system in response to allergenic substances. Histamine is also involved in sexual arousal.

The best sources of histidine are meat, chicken, fish, dairy products, rice, rye, and wheat. There is no recommended daily allowance for histidine, but it should be noted that balanced intake is important with this nutrient. Megadoses of histidine supplements have been reported to cause stress and emotional reactions, including anxiety. Also, high levels of histidine have been linked to schizophrenia, while low levels are associated with rheumatoid arthritis.

When Alanine Meets Histidine

As mentioned earlier, carnosine is a dipeptide, which simply means it is a combination of two amino acids. And, as is often the case, when two beneficial substances come together, the result is greater than the sum of its parts. In the case of carnosine, its two parent amino acids give it some unique capabilities. Here is a brief overview of carnosine's "resume":

- Carnosine protects proteins in the body from a damaging process known as glycation that leads to inflammation, disease, and aging. Protein damage is especially relevant to anyone with diabetes or insulin resistance, because high blood sugar levels are involved in glycation.

- As an antioxidant, carnosine quenches four harmful free radicals, including hydroxyl radicals, the most destructive of all, thereby shielding our cells, the lipids surrounding our cells, and our DNA, (deoxyribonucleic acid, the material that carries the "blueprint" for cell creation and reproduction) from damage.

- Carnosine revives aging cells, restores their youthful appearance, and increases their life span.

- Adequate supplies of carnosine allow the heart muscle to contract more efficiently by enhancing calcium response in the heart's cells.

- Studies with athletes show that carnosine reduces buildup of lactic acid, a potentially harmful byproduct of exercise.

- Carnosine protects brain cells from beta-amyloid deposits, substances that are linked to Alzheimer's disease.

- When certain processes involving cells and enzymes go into overdrive, as is the case with excess "stickiness" in blood platelets that can lead to life-threatening blood clots, carnosine is able to "down-regulate" the process, thereby decreasing stickiness. At the same time, carnosine can also "up-regulate" the same events when blood is too thin.

- Carnosine prevents a form of protein damage that contributes to wrinkles and loss of elasticity in the skin.

- Stomach ulcers can be prevented as well as healed with carnosine, which has also been shown to be effective at healing wounds on the skin's surface.

- Carnosine binds with heavy metals, such as iron, copper, and zinc, and removes them from the body, minimizing potential damage.

- Energy available to cells is enhanced by carnosine, which delivers essential fatty acids into cell membranes where they are utilized for fuel. It also protects these fatty acids from free-radical damage.

- Carnosine heals cataracts by renewing proteins in the eye's lens that have been rendered nonfunctional by processes that occur with aging.

It's important to understand that while many of these processes may seem irrelevant at first glance, all are involved in one way or another in the development of a variety of diseases and health concerns. For example, treating or preventing ulcers can reduce the risk of developing stomach cancer. Similarly, keeping blood flowing smoothly, via carnosine's ability to increase or decrease platelet stickiness, minimizes heart disease risk. And combating free-radical and gly - cation damage throughout the body is an important step in reducing the likelihood of various types of cancer and other diseases.

Understanding Illness

To understand how carnosine works, it is important to know that illness begins at the cellular level. Even though we are unaware of the minute changes that eventually lead to disease and aging, they are ongoing and ever present. The human body is a vast collection of cells, some 10 trillion of them. There are roughly 200 different types of cells, including specialized cells in the muscles, blood, brain, nerves, liver, and so on. Despite their microscopic size, human cells are quite complex. Structurally, a cell is like a soft plastic sack filled with a gel-like substance, as well as other, smaller plastic bags. The outermost plastic bag, which is known as the cell membrane, protects all of the contents of the cell, while the smaller "bags" are membranes that shield specific contents of the cell, such as the DNA (deoxyribonucleic acid), which contains the cell's job description and other information, and structures like mitochondria, where each cell's energy is produced.

Mitochondria
Structures within the cells that convert nutrients into energy, and perform other vital tasks.

The cells' protective membranes are made up of proteins, carbohydrates, and lipids or fats. Although the primary job of each membrane is to protect the cell, membranes are far from rigid. In fact, in order for cells to function properly, cell membranes must be semipermeable, with components that can move, change, and perform essential physiological roles while allowing cells to exchange information with one another and the environment.

Defects in membranes or their components, or damage to a cell's DNA, which contains the cell's "instruction manual," are responsible for many of the diseases we know today. These defects can be caused by unstable rogue molecules known as free radicals, but there are so many other things that can damage cells, including pollution, medications, chemicals in household cleaning products and dry cleaning fluids, pesticides and hormones in food, and the substances our bodies produce during stressful times, to name only a few.

Cells Are Not the End of the Story

Within each cell, there are tiny organelles known as mitochondria. Chemical reactions within the mitochondria create the energy that cells use to function. Equally important, the mitochondria serve as the cell's "gatekeeper," with the power to determine if a cell will live or die, so it is essential that these microscopic organs be kept healthy.

Like our cells, the mitochondria have their own protective membranes and their own DNA, separate from that found in the nucleus of each cell. When a cell's DNA is damaged by free radicals, antioxidants can help repair it, but the same is not true of mitochondrial DNA. Once this sort of damage occurs, the mitochondria weaken and die, creating a slowdown in many essential processes. So, good health requires keeping both the cell membrane *and* the mitochondrial membrane healthy and fully functioning.

Carnosine is especially good at providing support to membranes of both the cell and the mitochondria. These membranes consist largely of phospholipids, or polyunsaturated fatty acids. The standard American diet is typically low in "good" fats, such as the omega-3 fatty acids found in flaxseeds, flaxseed oil, and certain types of fish, and far too high in omega-6 fatty acids from a steady diet of fast and junk foods, snacks, and desserts made with vegetable oils. If the resulting imbalance is not corrected by supplementing with good fats, the membranes of our cells and mitochondria are especially vulnerable to damage.

DNA is made up of chromosomes, which contain our genes, with the "chemical codes" that create all the various proteins in our bodies. Carnosine also has the ability to protect our DNA and chromosomes from damage that can cause genetic codes, or "instructions," to go awry, and make faulty proteins. Since the proteins are used to make such essential substances as enzymes, it's easy to see how a defect in a digestive enzyme, for example, could lead to all sorts of other problems. Dutch researchers at the Institute of Human Genetics at Amsterdam's Free University tested a number of antioxidants—including vitamins C and E, carnosine, glutathione, and N-acetylcysteine (NAC)—to see which were effective at minimizing chromosome breakage. Only carnosine provided protection for these vitally important elements.

Chromosomes
Slender bodies in the cell nucleus where genes are located.

Carnosine Supports Other Antioxidants

The human body produces its own antioxidants, such as superoxide dismutase (SOD) but these can be damaged by free radicals and rendered useless. A new study from South Korea found that carnosine and two closely related substances were able to provide significant protection for SOD by scavenging free radicals and removing metals so it could function properly. Carnosine has also been teamed with the antioxidant mineral zinc as a remedy for stomach ulcers, something we'll look at in more detail in Chapter 6.

Obviously, carnosine can be a valuable addition to any antioxidant arsenal. By protecting our cellular and mitochondrial membranes, as well as chromosomes and DNA, carnosine prevents the chemical reactions that are at the very root of so many illnesses. In Chapter 4, we will learn more about carnosine's antioxidant abilities. But first, let's take a close look at how carnosine provides one of its most essential and impressive services—maintaining the integrity of the body's proteins, a little-understood advantage that can protect us against deterioration due to aging, as well as a wide range of illnesses.

CHAPTER 2

PROTECTING PROTEINS: CARNOSINE'S PRIMARY JOB

The free-radical theory of aging has had a great deal of exposure in both scientific and consumer publications. Less well known—but equally damaging—is a process known as glycation (sometimes referred to glycosylation). Glycation plays a major role in disease and aging, both internally and externally, because of its effect on proteins.

We have become accustomed to thinking of protein in terms of food because of the popularity of high-protein/low-carbohydrate diets. There is much more to the protein story, though. The body is primarily made of protein, and proteins are involved in most of its functions. These proteins change as we age, and they are exposed to damaging free radicals or different forms of sugar, which cause glycation. Like free radicals, glycation compromises proteins, robbing them of their ability to perform properly. When proteins malfunction, we become vulnerable to diseases, and ailments that are often considered part of the aging process are more likely to occur. Carnosine is one of the few substances with the special ability to ward off both free radicals and glycation. In Chapter 4, we will take a more in-depth look at free radicals and how carnosine neutralizes them. But first, let's con -

Proteins
Essential components of muscles, skin, bones, and the body as a whole.

The Father of Glycation

Discovered in 1912 by French scientist Louis Maillard, glycation is sometimes called the Maillard reaction.

---

sider glycation, the harmful process that occurs when sugars interact with protein, and how carnosine can minimize it.

How Sugar Harms Protein

Essentially, glycation turns healthy proteins into unhealthy substances through a process known as "cross-linking." A more familiar form of glycation occurs when meat is heated and turns brown. Although our bodies are not nearly as hot as ovens, essentially the same thing occurs, just much more slowly. What happens is this: A molecule of glucose, fructose, or another type of sugar binds to a protein molecule. In essence, this makes the protein "sticky," and it is now possible for the first protein molecule to bind with a second one, in a process known as "cross-linking." The eventual results are damaged, nonfunctional substances known as "advanced glycation end products" or AGEs.

Here's an analogy to help make the glycation process a little clearer: Let's say you are driving down the street, all systems go. Suddenly, the wheels of your car run into a patch of freshly poured cement and become mired in it. All the benefits of driving are gone. Not only are you unable to move, but you're also holding up traffic, and your car is actually now a hazard to other drivers. In other words, a formerly good, useful thing has become a liability.

Cross-linking causes the same thing to happen to proteins in the body. As we saw earlier, proteins are absolutely essential to life and are involved in many vital processes. But in order for them to function properly, they must remain independent of one another. Cross-linking, which fuses proteins together, renders them as useless as a car whose wheels are stuck in cement. And like the car, these cross-linked proteins, and especially the AGEs they spawn, can be dangerous. Glycated proteins produce damaging free radicals at an astonishingly high rate, as much as fifty times that of normal proteins!

To make matters worse, sugars can also cause protein to cross-link with the DNA that cells use to replicate themselves. The results can be disastrous, because cross-linked DNA can lead cells to make mistakes in the duplication process. In essence, these kinds of mistakes are like writing down a recipe incorrectly. If one ingredient or measurement is off, instead of ending up with muffins, for example, you could find yourself with a plateful of hardened dough balls that resemble hockey pucks.

When free radicals from glycated proteins damage cells, they can cause the same sort of errors. Instead of producing normal protein, a cell with defective instructions will produce abnormal proteins. Since the immune system's job is to identify and eliminate foreign "invaders," it may easily mistake the de - fective protein for an enemy and attack. If the assault continues, the result could be an autoimmune disease, cancer, or other serious health concern. As we will see shortly, carno-

Autoimmune Disease

An illness in which the body's tissues are attacked by its own immune system. Rheumatoid arthritis and systemic lupus erythematosus are two autoimmune diseases.

sine can help prevent the "hockey-puck muffin" scenario from occurring, with its ability to protect both protein and genetic coding from free-radical damage. But first, let's take a look at a few of the ways cross-linking affects health.

Cross-Linking: Hazardous to Your Health

An accumulation of cross-linked proteins can stiffen connective tissues and organs, leading to cardiovascular difficulties as well as joint problems. The AGEs that are produced by cross-linked proteins also affect everything from cell functions to mental abilities and vision. Here are some recent findings that clarify glycation's role in common diseases:

- British researchers concluded that cataracts, the leading cause of blindness worldwide, are a direct result of changes caused by glycation.

- Another study found that glycation is responsible for the stiff, brittle cartilage that causes painful joint diseases, such as osteoarthritis.

- Protein damage due to glycation was determined to be associated with brain neuron damage and other physiological changes found in Alzheimer's patients.

- Glycation plays a role in inflammation, which was recently identified as a risk factor for heart disease, stroke, and a host of other ailments.

- Scientists also know that glycation is linked to cancer, but they have not yet determined whether it is a cause or a result of tumor formation.

The dangers of glycation are all too familiar to anyone with diabetes. This disease increases glycation, and diabetics tend to age more quickly than those without the condition. Remember that diabetics may have high levels of blood glucose, which means there are more sugar molecules available for the glycation process. In Chapter 3, we will take a more in-depth look at carnosine's effect on diabetes and Syndrome X, an umbrella term for a condition characterized by insulin resist-

Insulin Resistance
The cells' inability to recognize and respond to insulin's attempts to transport sugar from the bloodstream into muscle and other tissues.

ance, excess weight (especially in the abdominal area), high blood pressure, and high blood levels of triglycerides.

Carnosine to the Rescue

Extensive studies have shown that carnosine is at the top of the list when it comes to preventing glycation. Not only is carnosine effective at interfering with the process, but it is also safe and free of side effects. In seven recent studies, for example, carnosine has proven to effectively protect various types of protein from common enemies, including fructose, formaldehyde, and malondialdehyde (MDA), a toxic byproduct created when fats in the bloodstream are oxidized.

Furthermore, according to a recent report in *Free Radicals in Biology and Medicine,* carnosine was able to inhibit cross-linking in oxidized proteins (i.e., those already converted to "enemies" by exposure to free radicals). Oxidized proteins can compromise healthy proteins, in the same way as their glycated cousins, but in this experiment, carnosine was found to be capable of rendering them harmless.

Smoother Skin with Carnosine

Pinch some skin together and it will pucker up

with wrinkles. Release it, and, like magic, they disappear. Proteins form the elasticlike collagen in our skin that makes this possible. When collagen formation slows during aging, our skin loses its flexibility and becomes thinner, with an almost papery appearance. Glycation causes the loss of collagen protein in the skin, which results in wrinkles. By interfering with the glycation process, carnosine can help minimize wrinkling when applied topically, and is now available in skin creams.

Collagen
The primary protein found in the skin, tendons, cartilage, bone, and connective tissue.

Internally, carnosine should strengthen collagen production, as well. And Australian scientists have shown that carnosine can do just that. They conducted landmark research showing that when aged human cells were treated with carnosine they recovered their youthful appearance and the number of times they could divide increased. Further studies at Sydney University determined that carnosine helps support the skin's immune defenses from damage by ultraviolet radiation caused by sun exposure.

Protecting the skin and keeping it healthy is not just a cosmetic concern. As the largest organ of our bodies, skin protects us from infection and dehydration. The outer layer of skin, known as the epidermis, is actually made up of dead cells. Our epidermis is constantly being renewed, as old, dead cells fall off and are replaced by new ones. But wrinkles settle deep into the dermis, the layer beneath the epidermis. Facial peels and similar techniques remove some of the outer layer of dead cells, giving the skin a fresh look, but it's temporary. Dermatologists are also concerned about the wrinkle-encouraging and cancer-promoting side effects of constantly ex -

posing a new layer of skin cells to sunlight, which is what occurs when we use lotions containing fruit acids on a regular basis.

Meanwhile, scientists have been busy developing "fillers" that can be injected into wrinkles to plump them up. Although there are a growing number of choices available today, the technique is not foolproof and all are temporary. Ideally, the best way to keep skin looking young is by increasing collagen formation by means of a natural method, such as carnosine.

Cut the Sugar

One way to reduce damaging protein cross-linking and the amount of AGEs in your body is to reduce the consumption of simple carbohydrates, like sugar. According to a recent study from Germany, foods containing fructose, a type of sugar found in fruit, are especially damaging. Researchers compared two groups of healthy subjects. One group ate a traditional diet, while the other adhered to a vegetarian-eating plan. They found that because vegetarians typically consumed less protein and more fruit than those who ate a traditional diet, they had a higher intake of fructose, which tends to be highly reactive and therefore more likely to form AGEs than the glucose derived from carbohydrates.

At first, these findings might seem confusing, considering the general wisdom that fruits and vegetables are healthy choices. But the researchers themselves help explain this seeming contradiction. The problem, they noted, is most fruits—and even some vegetables—contain more fructose than glucose. And fruit juices, which have little of fruit's beneficial fiber, are also loaded with fructose.

Although fruit is undoubtedly beneficial in

terms of providing antioxidants and fiber, the researchers noted that better choices would be those with the lowest levels of fructose. Generally, bitter or acidic fruits, like rhubarb and citrus, have low fructose content. On the other hand, carnosine can head off glycation, making it possible to have your fruit and eat it, too.

Fructose is not the only culprit involved in glycation. Experts believe that a ubiquitous "sweetener" known as high fructose corn syrup is playing a major role in the growing obesity epidemic, as well as other health problems. In Chapter 3, we will look at other ways carnosine can counteract the effects of sugar and high fructose corn syrup, while improving the health of people with diabetes and Syndrome X, aiding in blood sugar management, and helping control weight.

THE CARNOSINE CONNECTION TO DIABETES, SYNDROME X, AND WEIGHT MANAGEMENT

About 17 million individuals in this country live with diabetes, while untold millions of others suffer from a condition known as Syndrome X, a cluster of symptoms that includes excessive weight (especially around the abdomen), high blood pressure, and high levels of triglycerides in the bloodstream. In addition to these ailments, a recent survey in the *Journal of the American Medical Association* (*JAMA*) reported that the number of Americans who are overweight or obese is higher than ever, with 64.5 percent of the population now considered overweight or obese.

Overweight versus Obese
Overweight is defined as a body mass index (BMI) between 25 and 29.9. Obese individuals have a BMI of 30 or more.

For many people, a few extra pounds mean clothes that are a little too snug or a harder struggle to suck in the tummy. But the real danger of weight gain isn't cosmetic. Adding even one or two pounds a year can have serious health consequences.

The Price of Obesity

Roughly 300,000 Americans die each year as a result of obesity. Annually, more than half of all deaths in this country are caused by heart dis-

Inflammation
The body's reaction to infection, irritation, or other injury. Symp - toms include pain, redness, warmth, and/or swelling.

ease and cancer, and people who are obese have a higher likelihood of developing both. They are also at increased risk for diabetes and stroke, two other diseases that claim millions of lives each year.

In terms of weight gain, it doesn't take much to put one's health at risk. Fat churns out proteins that encourage inflammation, a condition that is now known to be linked to heart disease, stroke, and diabetes, as well as other health concerns.

Fat also produces hormones such as leptin, which has a complicated role in appetite management, and estrogen, a sex hormone that performs a host of necessary duties, but also has a downside: it is believed to play a role in the development of postmenopausal breast cancer. Abdominal fat, the kind commonly found in individuals with Syndrome X, seems to be the most *productive* in terms of creating these potentially damaging substances.

To see just how dangerous excess weight can be, we only need to look at one study of more than 120,000 middle-aged men and women, conducted at Brigham and Women's Hospital and Harvard Medical School. Health experts studying this group found that those with extra pounds had an increased risk of developing heart disease, high blood pressure, stroke, type 2 diabetes, colon cancer, and gallstones. The more overweight an individual was, the more likely he would be to develop multiple health problems. But even carrying a few additional pounds in - creased the risk of developing at least one chronic health condition.

How Weight Losers Win

Losing just a little weight can help a lot, though, say researchers. For example, trimming off 10 percent of one's body weight over a six-month period can reduce borderline high blood pressure and cut diabetes risk by nearly 60 percent. And weight management doesn't have to involve intensive, Olympic-style training or arduous exercise regimens. A Duke University Medical Center study, recently published in the *Archives of Internal Medicine*, found that a daily walk of 30 minutes was all it took to prevent the typical one- to two-pound weight gain that most adults expe - rience each year. Of course, a little more effort generated better results. Of the three groups observed in this eight-month-long study, the one that exercised vigorously (20 miles weekly jogging or riding a stationary bike, for example) shed 3.5 percent of body weight, compared to a 1 percent drop in the walking group. Still, if your goal is to merely stay where you are weight-wise, walking can do the trick. As we will see in Chapter 5, carnosine can provide muscles with the energy they need to perform harder and longer, which has additional advantages in terms of weight control and loss.

The Culture Connection

Unfortunately, weight gain has become an ac - cepted part of growing older. How often have you heard someone use the term "middle-age spread," for example, or talk about how much thinner they used to be when they were young? There is no doubt that our metabolism slows as we age, making weight gain more likely. But living in a nation of "super-sized," fast-food menus and restaurant portions that amount to two or more meals doesn't help either. At the same time, few people are active enough to burn off the steady high levels of calories they're taking in. While it's tempting to blame excess pounds on growing older, the truth is simply that weight is a lifestyle issue, and one that can be turned around.

Calorie
A unit of food energy. Comparing calories eaten to calories used in exercise is a reliable way to determine whether you are eating too much for your activity level.

In other words, the bottom line is that weight gain does not have to be an inevitable part of growing older. Whittling down serving sizes and increasing physical activity are the first line of defense against those extra pounds. Carnosine can help by making exercise more efficient and increasing muscle strength, thereby encouraging more calorie burning. (More on this later in Chapter 5.)

Another way to keep weight from piling up is by eating smarter. A good place to start that process is by staying away from sugar and simple carbohydrates—processed white flour, for example, found in bread, snacks, and pasta—because simple carbs are handled the same way as sugar in the body.

And be sure to watch portion sizes during mealtime. A 2004 report from the Centers for Disease Control and Prevention (CDC) found that Americans, and women in particular, are eating more than ever before. In 1971, a woman's average daily calorie intake was 1,542 calories. In 2000, that had soared to 1,877, a 22 percent increase! Men, by contrast, had only added an extra 7 percent to their daily intake during the same time period.

Furthermore, according to the CDC, most of those extra calories are coming from carbohydrates. While the survey didn't specify whether those carbs were simple or complex, other experts point to the increased consumption of soft drinks and snack foods during the same time period, and to the growing portion sizes in restaurants. As we have seen, various forms of sugar are responsible for protein-damaging glycation, which carnosine can combat. And one disease where glycation and excess weight play significant roles is type 2 (adult-onset) diabetes.

Diabetes: An American Epidemic

Type 2 diabetes is usually the result of a lifestyle that consists of too much food and not enough exercise. People who are diabetic do not produce enough insulin to properly manage their blood sugar levels. The number of people in this country with diabetes is growing at an alarming rate. Experts at the American Diabetes Association say that one in seven Americans, or nearly 30 million men and women, either have the disease or are on the verge of developing it, due to problems with blood sugar management. About 5 million of the 17 million individuals with diabetes do not even know they have it. Another 12.3 million are considered "pre-diabetic," meaning they are at risk of developing the disease during the next ten years.

Symptoms of diabetes include excessive thirst, increased frequency of urination, fatigue, hunger, weight loss, problems with vision, con-fusion or loss of consciousness, and pain or tingling sensations, especially in the feet or lower legs. Diabetes can lead to serious complications, including heart disease, blindness, circulatory problems, and damage to the kidneys, liver, and nerves. Vigilant monitoring of blood sugar levels decreases the risk of developing such health problems.

Although sugar does not cause diabetes, it certainly plays a role in weight gain and obesity, and those factors are undeniably linked to diabetes. Given that connection, it is not terribly surprising that a disease like diabetes is on the rise; the typical American consumes about 130 pounds of sugar a year—much of it unwittingly! Combine that with the fact that few of us exercise regularly (exercise helps by preventing weight gain, and by increasing insulin's efficiency in the body) and it's easy to see why health experts are concerned. Even children today are being diagnosed with type 2 diabetes, once known as adult-onset diabetes, at an alarming rate. (Type 1 diabetes, formerly known as "juvenile onset" diabetes, is actually an autoimmune disorder and is usually diagnosed during childhood or adolescence, while type 2 is related to lifestyle and normally occurs later in life.)

Sugar can affect the body's reaction to insulin. Scientists are finding that a steady diet of sugar, in all its many forms, can cause the liver to unleash stored fats into the bloodstream in the form of triglycerides. A heavy load of triglycerides can make muscle and fat cells resistant to insulin's effects. Even worse, when fat cells become insulin resistant, they can discharge fatty acids into the bloodstream that actually attack and kill the insulin-producing cells of the pancreas. The eventual outcome: type 2 diabetes.

Pancreas
A small organ behind the stomach that produces the hormone insulin, among its other functions.

Diabetes can be managed. By following a sensible diet and exercising moderately and regularly, many people with diabetes are able to live with the disease and do not require insulin injections to control blood sugar levels. However, it is important to take a responsible, proactive approach to diabetes because it can cause premature aging throughout the body. In fact, people with diabetes are more vulnerable to such common age-related conditions as cardiovascular disease.

Carnosine and Diabetes

Carnosine can help people with diabetes in several important ways. Excessive levels of blood sugar and poor blood sugar management result in the formation of advanced glycation end products (AGEs), substances that are not our friends. As we saw in Chapter 2, AGEs cause proteins to bond, which results in malfunctions that lead to illness. Also, AGEs form permanent clusters that produce high levels of damaging free radicals.

For diabetics, AGEs are a special problem. Because people with diabetes tend to have more glucose in the bloodstream, they also have more AGEs in their bodies. Since these substances can also cause large and small blood vessels throughout the body to deteriorate, they compromise the cardiovascular and circulatory systems, putting people with diabetes at risk for heart disease.

Antioxidants are not able to prevent AGEs from developing. In fact, researchers in Eastern Europe found that only a few substances can interfere with the AGE formation process, and carnosine is one of them. Not only is carnosine able to trap AGE precursors, but it also serves as an antioxidant, further reducing damage caused by the disease.

Here's another way carnosine can help people with diabetes: Two Russian experiments—one involving test-tube research, the other an animal study—demonstrated carnosine's ability to stabilize the membranes of red blood cells, which are prone to glycation in diabetics. Red blood cells are responsible for transporting oxygen to cells throughout the body. In people who do not have diabetes, only a very small percentage of red blood cells—usually about 5 percent—are glycated, and therefore unable to function. In diabetics, however, glycation can compromise as much as 25 percent of red blood cells. The researchers found that carnosine increased the number of healthy red blood cells in diabetic circumstances and protected them from glycation.

Avoiding Syndrome X

In the 1980s, Dr. Gerry Reaven, of Stanford University, coined the phrase "Syndrome X" to describe a cluster of symptoms that are also known as "metabolic syndrome." Syndrome X is a precursor to diabetes itself. People with Syndrome X often experience "insulin resistance," a condition in which insulin is being produced, but it is not recognized, so blood sugar levels remain high.

Insulin resistance is often accompanied by other factors that are detrimental to health, including high blood triglyceride levels, and low levels of "good," HDL cholesterol, obesity (especially when fat is primarily located in the abdomen), and high blood pressure. Together, these conditions are known as Syndrome X. Most often, Syndrome X is found in middle-aged people, where it is considered a risk factor for heart disease and other serious health issues. Experts believe that as many as 30 percent of the adults in countries where the "Western" lifestyle is common have Syndrome X, but few of them are aware of it. In this country alone, insulin resistance occurs

Triglycerides
A common form of fat found in the blood-stream.

in varying degrees in as many as 70 million people.

Several groups of people are more likely than others to develop Syndrome X, according to the American Heart Association. They are: 1) anyone with high blood pressure who also has high levels of insulin; 2) diabetics with poor glucose tolerance; and 3) survivors of heart attacks who have high insulin levels.

When it comes to preventing or managing Syndrome X, scientists have discovered that there are steps you can take that can help. Avoiding simple carbohydrates, such as sugar, is one of them, because sugar is turning out to be just as damaging as saturated fat, in terms of its effect on our health. But avoiding such simple carbohydrates is easier said than done. Sugar, in a variety of guises, is everywhere, including some very unlikely foods. To make matters worse, a chemically manufactured sweetener known as high fructose corn syrup (HFCS) is widely used in food manufacturing today, with what many experts believe to be disastrous results. But with a little effort, you can avoid sugar in its different forms— once you know what to look for.

Why Sugar Is Not So Sweet

Given our national obsession with fat—and the corresponding surge in the number of low-fat foods available—one might think that heart disease, diabetes, and Syndrome X are on their way to becoming history. Of course, this is far from the case. Heart disease is still the nation's number-one killer, and the rates of obesity and diabetes are soaring. Meanwhile, Americans are spending billions of dollars on low-fat foods, not to mention weight-loss products, with nothing but frustration to show for their investment.

Part of the problem, say some health experts, is that too much low-fat fare is actually loaded with calories. How can this be? Because very often food manufacturers have increased sugar content to improve the flavor of these products.

A trip down the aisle of any grocery store will provide dozens of illustrations. Ignore for a moment the colorful banners on food packaging declaring the contents to be "low-fat" or "fat free." Instead, compare the number of calories on one of these packages with the calories on a similar product that is not reduced in fat. Typically, the low-fat foods contain the same—or in some cases, more!—calories than the original version. In nearly every case, that's because the sugar content is higher.

When health experts began pointing this out to an unsuspecting public a few years ago, food manufacturers resorted to a sneaky new tactic. They manipulated the serving size on products, so that calorie content appeared lower on low-fat, high-sugar fare. In other words, consumers who looked at calorie content alone could miss the fact that the reason the low-fat cookies only had half as many calories as the regular version was because the serving size of the low-fat cookies was smaller.

Food manufacturers know that most of us do not have the time to study the fine print on product labels and do complicated ingredient comparisons. So they emblazon enticing phrases on packaging—such as "only $\frac{1}{2}$ gram of fat per serving"—to convince us that these foods are healthy. The truth, however, lies in the fine print. Invest in your health by spending a little time getting to know which products are actually good for you. (Hint: Almost all snacks, as well as ready-made and prepackaged foods—no matter how healthy they sound—are not good choices. The exceptions are those found in health-food stores, and even there, it pays to read the fine print.)

The Hidden Dangers of High-Fructose Corn Syrup

As you have probably noticed, trans fats have been the subject of a great deal of media attention recently. Found largely in foods made with partially hydrogenated vegetable oils, these fats have been linked to heart disease and other health concerns, but have never been listed on nutrition labels. Experts now say there appears to be no safe level of trans fat intake. As a result, the Food and Drug Administration (FDA) has ordered food manufacturers to include the amount of trans fats on food labels by 2006. This is all well and good. But many health experts are wondering how high-fructose corn syrup (HFCS), an equally dangerous dietary villain, has managed to slip under the radar.

Why is HFCS so bad? Experts say there are three factors involved. One, the body does not absorb fructose the same way as other sugars. For example, HFCS does not stimulate production of insulin, the hormone that enables sugar to be delivered to the cells to provide energy. Nor does it have any effect on two other appetite-regulating hormones, leptin and ghrelin. These differences are important, because they mean consuming HFCS does not satisfy hunger pangs the way a sugar like sucrose or glucose does. The bottom line: HFCS contributes to weight gain and obesity.

Not convinced? Consider these statistics—in 1966, the most commonly used sugar in this country was sucrose, which is simply another name for white, refined "table" sugar. At that time, sucrose so dominated the market that it accounted for nearly 90 percent of sweeteners used in our food. In fact, that same year, no HFCS was consumed. Today, the situation is drastically different. Corn sweeteners make up more than half the sugar market, and the average American takes in more than 62 pounds of corn sweeteners a year! At the same time that our consumption of HFCS has been rising, Americans have been growing steadily heavier. You don't have to be a rocket scientist to see the connection between HFCS and obesity.

Sucrose
A disaccharide made up of glu - cose and fructose; "table sugar."

But weight isn't the only health concern related to HFCS. In a study at the University of Minnesota, researchers compared the effects of two different diets on a group of healthy adults. In one diet, 17 percent of the calories came from fructose, while the other consisted primarily of glucose, with almost no fructose. Otherwise, the diets were almost identical. At the end of the study, triglyceride levels in the men on the high fructose diet had soared by 32 percent. A similar study involving animals had the same results. High triglycerides are a major factor in cardiovascular disease, the nation's leading cause of death.

Another study, this one conducted in Hono - lulu, Hawaii, found liver dysfunction in healthy young men just five days after starting a fructose-rich diet. And a different team of researchers in Honolulu created quite a stir recently when they announced finding a link between fruit and fruit-drink consumption and Parkinson's disease, a neurodegenerative disease affecting nearly 2 million Americans. Their study, presented at a recent annual meeting of the American Academy of

Neurology, involved more than 8,000 men and women, with data collected for the previous thirty-four years. It found a clear connection between high consumption of fruit and fruit drinks and Parkinson's. While the study authors speculated it could be due to pesticides, herbicides, or other plant-related toxins, other experts point to the considerable amounts of HFCS added to fruit drinks as a possible culprit. It's interesting to note that scientists are finding that carnosine is showing promise as a weapon against Parkinson's, something we will look at further in Chapter 7.

An Unnatural Sugar

With links to both obesity and heart disease, it would seem that HFCS would be the focus of health warnings and possible legislation. Unfortunately, corn sweeteners are cheap, easier to use than other types of sugar, and very tasty—all factors that are appealing to food manufacturers. Add to this the fact that even a watchful consumer can be misled into thinking that these products are perfectly safe, simply because they seem so harmless. After all, how can corn be bad for us?

But the truth is HFCS is a far cry from actual corn or even that old standby, corn syrup, which is mainly glucose. HFCS is a mass-produced, chemical creation of technological wizardry, with nearly limitless applications. Food processors use it because it enhances certain desirable qualities, like moisture and flavor. But the downside is that HFCS has a high amount of fructose—nearly 15 percent—far more than any food found in nature.

As we have seen, because of the way our bodies metabolize HFCS, it should not be part of a healthy diet. But just try eliminating it from your pantry! HFCS is found in hundreds of foods, including soft drinks, fruit beverages, ice cream, chewing gum, bread and other baked goods, jam and jelly, and countless other products, including such unlikely suspects as salad dressing and ketchup.

Weight gain, liver malfunction, high triglycerides, and Parkinson's disease aren't the only health problems associated with fructose and HFCS. Experts estimate that a fairly sizable number of Americans are fructose-intolerant. For them, even the small amount of HFCS that is typically found in a soda—about 25 grams—can cause stomach cramps, diarrhea, gas, and bloating. Some people are so fructose-intolerant that they can't absorb even tiny amounts of HFCS; they experience serious digestive distress from large quantities. Ironically, HFCS is also widely used in products aimed at athletes, like sport drinks, and energy and protein bars, and may undermine an exerciser's weight-management efforts.

If you would like to eliminate HFCS from your diet, here are a few suggestions. First, give up soft drinks, and trade apple juice (which often contains HFCS as well as a considerable amount of fructose) for a lower-fructose drink. Check food labels and avoid as many products as possible that contain 8 or more grams of any kind of sugar. Also, pass on foods with HFCS listed as the first or second ingredient. Cereals that may appear healthy, for example, are often loaded with HFCS. Even yogurt can be sweetened with this less-than-desirable substance.

Eliminating as much sugar and HFCS from your diet as possible is a major step toward better health and slower aging. Not only are you avoiding the empty calories these products contain, but you're also helping your digestive system work more efficiently, which translates into better overall health. Just as important, cutting back on various forms of sugar also reduces the amount of glycation taking place in your body, so you'll be fighting aging at the same time. And of course, as we saw earlier in the chapter, carnosine, an important weapon against glycation and aging in general, can help, too.

All about Syndrome X

We have all heard about the importance of a healthy, nutritious diet and regular, moderate exercise when it comes to staying healthy. In fact, most of us have heard it so often that the words are nearly meaningless. Only after a health crisis occurs do we fully comprehend the importance of lifestyle. Faced with the possibility of a second heart attack, surgery, or other serious event, many people are inspired to "shape up." Suddenly, they find the time to cook vegetables and choose to replace red meat with fish or skinless chicken. They start walking, lose weight, and find themselves feeling better than they have in years. Many times, they wonder why they didn't do these things long ago.

If you find yourself frustrated by weight gain and saddled with high blood pressure, high levels of triglycerides, and LDL cholesterol, as well as problems with blood sugar management, consider it a wake up call. By making a few lifestyle changes, you can turn your health around.

A new study, reported in the *Archives of Internal Medicine,* offers a perfect example. Research - ers at Duke University Medical Center found that a combination of exercise and weight loss dramatically lowered excess insulin pro duction and blood pressure in a group of people diagnosed with Syndrome X. Insulin production dropped by nearly 50 percent in the exercise–weight loss group, and even fell by 27 percent in a second group of individuals who exercised but did not lose weight.

Of course, most people have experienced the muscle aches and soreness that follow the first day's workout. Those pains are caused by lactic acid, a byproduct of muscle use.

Muscle cells make lactic acid when they use glucose (sugar) for energy. Some people experience sore muscles the day after a hard workout, or if they haven't exercised in a while. But if too much lactic acid stays in the body, a person can become ill. The signs of lactic acidosis are deep and rapid breathing, vomiting, and abdominal pain.

Lactic Acidosis
A condition caused by the buildup of lactic acid in the body.

Lactic acidosis may be caused by diabetic ketoacidosis or liver or kidney disease. If you experience more than ordinary muscle soreness, check with your doctor.

Ordinary aches and pains, however, are simply signs that your muscles are being used. The minerals calcium and magnesium can ease this soreness. And as you become increasingly fit, carnosine may be helpful, because it makes muscles more efficient and able to work harder.

Overcoming Syndrome X

If you feel it's time to make some changes, get your physician's okay and follow these guidelines:

- Aim to lose weight by exercising daily and cutting back on saturated fats and foods high in sugar and simple carbohydrates.

- Eat more fiber (25 to 30 grams daily).

- Eat more fish, poultry, and beans to increase protein intake without adding fat.

- Exchange simple carbohydrates, like white bread and rice, for the complex versions, such as whole-wheat bread and brown rice.

- Try to avoid constant snacking, which causes the liver to produce a steady stream of fat.

In addition, carnosine supplements can help strengthen muscles and make exercising more efficient, while improving health in many other ways. Earlier, we mentioned that free radicals play an important role in overall health and aging. Now it's time to see how carnosine combats those substances and protects us from harm.

CHAPTER 4

CARNOSINE AND FREE RADICALS, THE ENEMIES OF GOOD HEALTH

Once considered a topic of "fringe" medicine, the free-radical theory of aging is widely accepted today. Free radicals affect our health all throughout life and are believed to be responsible for a considerable number of health concerns, including the aging process. Technically speaking, free radicals are atoms or molecules with an unpaired electron. This electron shortage makes the atom or molecule unstable, so it tries to steal an electron from another atom or molecule. When the operation is a success, the theft creates a newly destabilized atom/molecule in search of an electron, and this destructive process begins all over again. Free radicals are such highly volatile substances that they last less than one-millionth of a second. Unfortunately, in that short span of time, they can do considerable damage.

> **Free Radicals**
> Atoms or molecules with an unpaired electron.

It's easiest to understand free radicals' impact on health with an analogy. Imagine, for example, that you have built a chair with the usual four legs. Then someone comes along and steals one of your chair's legs to build his own chair. The stolen leg is longer than his chair's other legs, though, and makes his chair tilt so sharply that it's no longer useful. Of course, your chair is no longer fully functional, either.

This may seem like a silly story, but it illustrates

in a simplified way how free radicals operate. Like the person who makes off with one of your chair's legs, a free radical steals another molecule's "leg," or, in this case, an electron. Destabilized by the loss, that molecule no longer functions properly, and neither does the new pair.

Free radicals vary greatly. Some are individual atoms, while others are clusters of atoms, or molecules. There are also different types of free radicals, including both good and bad. Good free radicals are absolutely essential to our health. They fortify the immune system by eliminating viruses and bacteria. They also stimulate the creation of essential enzymes, hormones, and other substances.

Other free radicals are not nearly so benign. Ironically, oxygen, the very substance we cannot live without, also has a downside. Among the most damaging and ubiquitous of all free radicals are those caused by oxidation, a process

Oxidation
A chemical reaction involved in digestion, burning, and rusting in which oxygen combines with another substance and electrons move between atoms.

that occurs when oxygen combines with another substance. In other words, every time we take a breath, free radicals are created. Hydrogen peroxide, nitric oxide, and lipid peroxides, which lead to artery-clogging deposits of fats and cholesterol, are only a few of the byproducts generated by the oxidizing process.

Free radicals were no doubt far less of a threat to the health of our Stone-Age ancestors. Why? Because modern life is filled with so many more sources of these damaging substances. Pollution, for example, didn't exist until very recently. Nor did the toxins found in today's household cleaning products, building materials, and chemicals in foods. Processed foods and high-fat diets are also fairly new occurrences and ones that put free-radical production into high gear simply because fat oxidizes more easily than either carbohydrates or protein. Frying and other methods of cooking that involve heating fat to high temperatures also boost free-radical numbers. (In Chapter 8, we will look at new research showing why foods cooked at extreme temperatures are unhealthy, and how carnosine can help minimize these dangers.)

Even things that are good for us can create free radicals. Since oxygen plays an important role in digestion, eating creates free radicals. And in a recent issue of the *Proceedings of the National Academy of Science*, Israeli researchers announced that they had discovered strenuous exercise leads to a flood of free radicals, far more than can be eliminated by the body's own defense mechanisms. Before heading for the couch, though, remember that exercise has too many benefits to use free radicals as an excuse not to work out. There are a number of substances that combat free radicals, including carnosine, which we will talk about shortly. But first, let's get an in-depth look at how free radicals affect health.

How Free Radicals Damage Health

Since the average person isn't likely to have an opportunity to observe cellular activity and the effect free radicals can have at microscopic levels, it's hard to imagine that these tiny, short-lived rogue molecules are actually harmful. So let's look at some actual examples of the damage caused by free radicals.

Heart attacks and strokes, two of the nation's leading killers, are frequently caused by atherosclerosis, or hardening of the arteries. Hardening of the arteries is a process that occurs over time, and eventually blocks blood flow to either the heart or brain. Arteries are "hardened" by deposits of fatty substances like cholesterol, especially low-density lipoprotein (LDL), or "bad" cholesterol. (Actually, LDL cholesterol does not start out "bad." In fact, it actually serves an important purpose—transporting fat-soluble vitamins and other

Atherosclerosis
A process that pro-gressively thickens and hardens the walls of arteries by depositing fat on their inner lining.

nutrients throughout the body. It is only after free radicals cause oxidization to occur that LDL cholesterol becomes the enemy.)

Hardening of the arteries may be easier to understand if you think of arteries as rubber tubes. Healthy arteries have some flexibility and can expand to allow small clusters of blood platelets to pass through. When fatty deposits collect on the inside of a tube, however, the tube not only loses its flexibility, but also becomes narrower. Small clumps of blood platelets may still manage to flow through the tube, but if these clumps grow larger and turn into a blood clot, they can obstruct the tube completely. When blood can no longer reach the heart, a heart attack occurs.

Free radicals play significant roles in hardening of the arteries as well as in the development of blood clots. In both cases, oxidation is to blame. Oxidized LDL cholesterol is one factor.

The Father of the Free-Radical Theory of Aging

Denham Harman, M.D., Ph.D., developed the free-radical theory of aging more than fifty years ago, while he was a professor at the University of California at Berkeley. It took years for his theory to become widely accepted.

Also, the process of oxidation makes blood platelets "stickier," so they tend to cluster together, eventually massing into clots.

Antioxidants Fight Free Radicals

Antioxidants combat oxidation. These are substances that combine with unstable free radicals before they can damage healthy cells. Free radicals are unavoidable. Even if we lived in a world without pollution, chemicals, and toxins, free radicals would still be part of our daily lives. Mother Nature equipped us to deal with a certain amount of these substances. Our bodies produce antioxidant compounds that counteract free radicals by donating an electron to these roguish, "three-legged chair" molecules and converting them into a stable, harmless, complete "chair."

Antioxidant
A substance that has the ability to counteract free-radical damage.

There are hundreds of antioxidant substances. Glutathione and superoxide dismutase (SOD), which our bodies can make, are two of the most important ones. Unfortunately, production of many of these essential substances slows as we age. Of course, we can also get antioxidants from foods, especially fruits and vegetables.

The Antioxidant Hall of Fame

In the past few years, researchers have discovered some extraordinary health benefits associated with popular antioxidants—vitamins A, C, and E, and the mineral selenium. They have also found powerful antioxidants in some lesser-known substances, such as alpha-lipoic acid (ALA), coenzyme Q_{10} (coQ_{10}), grape seed extract, N-acetylcysteine (NAC), the hormone melatonin, zinc, and plant pigments known as carotenoids and flavonoids.

Most of these nutrients have an affinity for a specific type of free radical. Vitamin A, for example, targets only one type—singlet oxygen—and ignores others. Obviously, the best free-radical protection is provided by a wide range of antioxidants, which is what we would get if we ate a nutritious, varied diet, including plenty of assorted fruits and vegetables that were grown in nutrient-rich soil. To get the same effect from supplements, we need to take more than one or two antioxidants. In fact, we need an array of these substances, so they can interact and support one another, just as Mother Nature intended.

Although it is not as well known as some other antioxidants, carnosine has impressive free-radical fighting abilities. Russian researchers have shown that carnosine tames not only the notoriously harmful hydroxyl free radicals, but peroxyl, singlet oxygen, and superoxide radicals as well. It is especially effective at protecting the brain's nerve cells. Scientists have noted that the amount of carnosine needed to spare these cells from free-radical damage was similar to, or even less than, what is typically found in the brain. Since carnosine levels throughout the body tend to diminish as we grow older, maintaining a sufficient supply of this nutrient could ward off much of the deterioration that is typically considered part of the aging process.

Carnosine also "plays well with others" by supporting the free-radical quenching activities of other antioxidants, especially the mineral zinc. Recently, zinc has gained attention for studies showing it can shorten the duration of the common cold. This is still somewhat controversial, but

Zinc
An essential mineral that is involved in the manufacture of protein and in cell division.

there is no doubt that this mineral plays a role in good health. Zinc is a recognized immune booster, with the ability to help the body repair wounds, create protein, and stimulate cell production. Zinc is also necessary for eye health. (In Chapter 6 we'll look at the synergistic effect of combining carnosine and zinc in treating stomach ulcers.)

Carnosine also serves as a barrier against free radicals for cell membranes as well as for the protective membrane around the mitochondria, the "energy factories" within each cell. Both types of membranes are vitally important. If a cell membrane is damaged, it no longer functions, and if the mitochondria's membrane is harmed, energy production ceases. Although there are billions of cells in our bodies, and each one has more than 1,000 mitochondria, when free-radical damage accumulates, we become vulnerable to a host of diseases, not to mention the aging process.

Free Radicals, Inflammation, and Carnosine

Inflammation is another serious consequence of unchecked free-radical activity, but again, it is one that carnosine can combat. Our diet and lifestyle has put us at risk for chronic low-grade inflammation. Until recently, inflammation's central role in illness and disease was not acknowledged. Only in the last few years have scientists begun to realize that inflammation plays a role in heart disease, arthritis, diabetes, allergies, Alzheimer's disease, obesity, asthma, ulcers, gum disease, and certain types of cancer.

Like so many natural processes, inflammation is not inherently bad. In fact, it is designed to help us survive. When you accidentally hit your finger with a hammer or sprain your ankle, the injured area swells and feels warm or tender to the touch. This is because the body rises to the occasion by initiating a process designed to dispose of damaged cells and create new re - placement cells. This sort of acute inflammation disappears after the area heals.

Similarly, whenever the skin is broken, there is a possibility that dangerous bacteria could enter the body. You may have noticed that even a wound as small as a paper cut turns red and swells slightly. That's a sign that your white blood cells, the body's first line of defense against harmful invaders, have arrived at the site, ready to do battle.

What's the difference between these types of "good" inflammation and the "bad" variety? The two examples above are acute, short-term solutions to temporary problems. The hammered finger and sprained ankle heal in a matter of days or weeks. The paper cut disappears within days. By contrast, inflammation becomes a problem when it turns into a chronic condition. Joints swollen by osteoarthritis are a common example. Millions of people suffer from this disabling disease, which is characterized by inflammation of the tissue surrounding the joints. A less visible, but potentially more lethal, form of chronic inflammation occurs in cardiovascular disease, as the walls of blood vessels become inflamed. Here, again, white blood cells are dispatched to quell the inflammation, but this process produces free radicals that only make the situation worse.

Osteo-arthritis
A type of arthritis caused by inflammation, degradation, and eventual loss of joint cartilage.

Conventional medicine treats inflammation with nonsteroidal, anti-inflammatory drugs (NSAIDs), such as aspirin, ibuprofen, and similar prescription medications, now a multibillion-dollar industry. And while these drugs do reduce inflammation temporarily, they can have serious side effects, including internal bleeding and death.

Fortunately, carnosine fights inflammation without the side effects associated with NSAIDs. It does this in two ways: First, because it is an active antioxidant, carnosine decreases the number of inflammation-producing free radicals in the body. Second, carnosine prevents glycation, the protein-damaging process we learned about in Chapter 2, which is also linked to inflammation.

Two recent studies show just how useful carnosine can be at inhibiting inflammation. The first study, conducted in Japan, found that a combination of carnosine and zinc was as effective at reducing inflammation of the colon in test animals as a commonly prescribed drug (sulfasalazine). In the second study, carnosine was found effective at preventing glycation of both normal and denatured protein, a type that often occurs at inflammation sites, leading researchers to speculate that carnosine's ability to inhibit glycation in two kinds of protein may be responsible for its anti-inflammatory properties.

Although good health is the result of many different factors, combating free radicals is a vitally important element. These abundant predators undermine health at its most basic level and set the stage for serious illness. Fortunately, anti-oxidants, including carnosine, can repair much of this damage.

CHAPTER 5

CARNOSINE FOR LONGEVITY

Aging is a complex process that affects us in many different ways. For some people, growing older means living with the discomfort of a joint disease, like osteoarthritis. For others, it could translate into weight gain, type 2 diabetes, osteoporosis, difficulties with vision or hearing, or all of the above. Once believed to be as inevitable as the passing of time, aging is the subject of a great deal of study today, as researchers attempt to extend life span and increase the number of active, healthy years at the same time.

Some of the most exciting news related to carnosine and longevity comes from Russia, where scientists have been studying the compound since its discovery in 1900. Researchers there recently discovered that supplemental carnosine could extend the life span of male fruit flies (*Drosophila melanogaster*) to match that of their long-lived female counterparts. The experts speculated that carnosine provided protection against age-related damage by free radicals.

"Why study fruit flies?" you may be asking. The simple answer is because their life span is so short—usually no more than a day—that results can be seen quickly. By the same token, longevity studies with longer-lived species, such as rats, take several years to obtain results. Clearly, it is almost impossible to study the effect of supplements on aging in humans. Such research would take several generations, so science draws con-clusions from clinical trials with other species and applies those conclusions to humans.

If you still have doubts about whether or not these studies are valid, take heart from a recent report in *Current Opinions in Neurology,* which was coauthored by experts at Brigham and Women's Hospital and Harvard Medical School. They noted the many contributions made to our knowledge of neurodegenerative disorders, like Parkinson's disease and Alzheimer's, by studies involving *Drosophila.*

There was one other notable finding in the study mentioned above. You may recall that ear-lier we discussed the fact that the synergy that occurs when alanine and histidine combine gives carnosine greater potential than either of its components has individually. The Russian scien-tists found that to be the case: individual supple-ments of alanine and histidine did not have the same beneficial effect on life span as carnosine.

Several other studies have confirmed carno-sine's synergistic superiority over its individual elements. For example, British researchers noted that carnosine supplements improved appear-ance and physical condition of subjects in an ani-mal study. By comparison, a group that was given separate supplements of alanine and histidine did not show the same improvements.

Another milestone in carnosine research was reported by scientists at Moscow State University who compared the effects of carnosine on two groups of mice—one normal, and the other "senescence-accelerated mice" (SAM), which have been bred to age more quickly than the norm.

In the SAM group, carnosine prevented the development of physical and behavioral signs of senility, and also increased average life span.

Carnosine had a similar effect on the normal mice, but it was less noticeable because this group aged more slowly. Given what we know about the similarities between mice and humans—which is actually a great deal—there is no reason to think carnosine would not have the same anti-aging effect on people.

Live Long, Live Strong

One thing research is making clear is the role of lifestyle in aging. There is little doubt, for example, that lack of exercise and the less-than-nutritious diet so many Americans consume contributes to the overall decline associated with aging. Exercise is especially important, say many authorities, and because of carnosine's intimate relationship with muscle tissue, it is an ideal supplement for anyone who wants to age well.

As we learned earlier, the highest concentrations of carnosine are found in the muscles, particularly in the heart and skeletal muscle tissues. Skeletal, or voluntary, muscles are attached to our bones with tendons, so we can move them at will. We have more than 650 voluntary muscles in our bodies. The amount of carnosine in the muscles is considered a potential biomarker of life span. In other words, say health experts, the more carnosine in the muscles, the longer one is likely to live.

Beyond Bones

Osteoporosis has received a great deal of attention in recent years. There is no doubt that osteoporosis is both serious and widespread—experts say as many as 25 million women and men may suffer from the condition. This debilitating and

Osteoporosis
Thinning of the bones with reduction in bone mass due to reduction of calcium and bone protein.

frequently painful condition is responsible for the brittle bones that can break during a fall and are slow to heal, leading to further complications.

But osteoporosis is only part of the story. A less well-known but equally serious condition, sarcopenia (pronounced "sar-ko-PEEN-ya") is only beginning to get the attention it deserves. Just as osteoporosis is considered a bone-thinning disease, sarcopenia could be called a "muscle-thinning" disease. After age forty, adults lose one-quarter to one-third of a pound of muscle a year and gain that much body fat. Lean muscle, which is one of the leading calorie burners in the body, starts to erode in early adulthood. By middle age, the process is well underway, and loss of muscle is the greatest single factor in the increasing accumulation of excess body fat. Muscle tissue lost during aging, and often replaced with fat, increases the likelihood of falls and broken bones in the elderly. This loss of muscle has been labeled sarcopenia.

Muscle
Tissue that functions primarily as a source of power. The three types of muscle are skeletal muscle, which moves our limbs, cardiac muscle in the heart, and smooth muscle in artery walls and in the bowel.

Ironically, our national obsession with weight loss is actually a major contributing factor to weight gain and many of the detrimental effects of aging. Here's why: When the body is deprived of nutrition—say, a skipped breakfast, for example, or even a hearty lunch of processed, nutrition-free junk food—it goes to its emergency reserves, which are stored in lean muscle tissue.

As the amount of muscle tissue in the body decreases, so do the number of calories burned at rest. So the body is burning off less of the food that is eaten and the muscles are weakened, making muscle-building, strenuous exercise less likely. Weight gain occurs. Dieting begins. The body is getting even less nutrition, and so it devours more muscle tissue. This vicious cycle of muscle loss and weight gain can continue indefinitely, with disastrous results. As muscles weaken, body fat continues to accumulate, and the combination eventually interferes with an individual's ability to perform everyday tasks.

Two recent studies illustrate the connections among aging, low levels of carnosine, and weight gain. First, researchers in England compared carnosine levels in the muscles of both young (about twenty-four years old) and older (about seventy years old) subjects. They found the older individuals had significantly less carnosine in their muscles, leading these experts to conclude that sarcopenia was responsible for the wide difference in carnosine levels.

In the second study, conducted at Pennsylvania State University with nearly 3,000 men and women aged seventy or older, researchers found that women with the highest percentage of body fat were twice as likely to report limitations in their ability to carry out normal everyday living tasks, such as carrying a 10-pound grocery bag. Men fared somewhat better, with those with the greatest percentage of body fat 1.5 times more likely to report difficulty functioning on a daily basis. Clearly, aging well requires weight management and muscle maintenance, and carnosine excels in both.

Building a Better Body

There is considerable research showing that exercise has enormous benefits, especially for older adults, in terms of both physical and mental health. Regular workouts reduce or prevent many age-related illnesses, including heart disease, arthritis, osteoporosis, diabetes, obesity, and depression. As one expert noted, if exercise came in pill form, it would be the top-selling medication in the world.

Between the ages of ten and seventy, the levels of carnosine in our muscles plummet by 60 percent or more. Carnosine supplements, however, can prevent this. In addition, they can help keep us fit by making our muscles more efficient when we exercise. In Japan, where there is great interest in carnosine, researchers recently found that the amount of carnosine in the muscles of healthy men was associated with power during a thirty-second sprint, especially during the last two five-second intervals. As the experts noted, "These results indicated that the carnosine concentration could be an important factor in determining the high-intensity exercise performance."

In Italy, scientists found yet another beneficial link between carnosine and exercise. As we mentioned in Chapter 4, free radicals are a natural byproduct of physical activity. But results of a clinical trial at the University of Milan showed that carnosine significantly reduced the free radicals generated by exercise.

Another potential benefit of carnosine lies in preventing age-related neuromuscular diseases, such as polymyositis, an autoimmune disorder involving inflammation of the muscle tissue, and the degenerative condition known as Lou Gehrig's disease (amyotrophic lateral sclerosis, or ALS). As German scientists at the University Hospital in Hamburg-Eppendorf noted, aging muscles are increasingly vulnerable to such diseases, and this is especially true for anyone with a genetic predisposition due to a family history of such illnesses. They also observed that carnosine could alter the physical effects that aging has on muscles, as well as shield muscles from free-radical damage that is related to some of these disorders.

Move It or Lose It

If you've been sedentary and are now inspired to start working out, congratulations! Keep in mind, though, that it's important to get your physician's approval before starting an exercise program. After getting the go-ahead, use the slow but steady approach to avoid injury. Experts advise setting realistic, short-term goals, ideally with the help of a trainer or by enrolling in a beginner's class at the health club or local YMCA/YWCA.

Also, remember that while aerobic exercise is excellent for strengthening the cardiovascular system and for burning calories, weight training is especially important for maintaining muscles, which in turn burn calories. You don't need any fancy equipment to accomplish this goal; small free-weights or even inexpensive resistance bands, large rubber bands designed for work - outs, will do the job. But keep a couple of things in mind. One, the type of weight training we are talking about will not bulk you up or make you look like a contender in a bodybuilding competition. Many women are especially hesitant to begin a weight-training routine because they are concerned about excessive muscle development. It simply will not happen. Bodybuilders go to extreme lengths to achieve those results, involving far more drastic measures than the average person is willing to endure. Fortunately, working out with free weights, or even

Aerobic Exercise
Brisk physical activity that requires the heart and lungs to work harder to meet the body's demands for increased oxygen.

ordinary weight-training equipment in a gym, for thirty or forty minutes three to five times a week will not create those results, but it will give you the strength to grow old gracefully and in good health.

Try Isometric Muscle Building

"Isometric exercise" is an exercise that involves tensing a muscle without moving a body part and holding the tension for six to eight seconds, then releasing and repeating five to ten times. ("Isotonic exercise," on the other hand, is an exercise that involves contracting muscles against a steady load, as in weight lifting.)

Isometric exercises are helpful for anyone recovering from injuries that limit range of motion, because arms and legs remain in place while only the muscles move.

Remember that muscle tissue weighs more than fat, so don't expect immediate results in terms of weight loss. As your muscles grow, however, you should see areas where fat typically collected—the thighs, or waist/tummy, for example—becoming reshaped as fat is replaced by muscle. Remember that workouts are not a license to go overboard at mealtime. If you eat a reasonably sensible diet and exercise, the extra calories burned by your growing muscles will translate into reasonable weight loss over time, which is how it should be. You did not gain 30, 40, or 50 pounds in a week, so don't expect to lose them quickly, either.

Keeping Cells Young

When it comes to longevity, carnosine affects more than muscles. Throughout life, our cells divide somewhere between twenty and thirty times. This continual cellular expansion is what makes a child grow into an adult. Once we reach adulthood, cell division slows. Eventually, because of their inherent limits, our cells are no longer able to divide.

Some forty years ago, Dr. Leonard Hayflick, of Stanford University, discovered the limits to human cell division, so the "Hayflick limit" is the term used to describe the finite number of times cell division can take place before a form of cellular suicide known as apoptosis occurs. So even though we need new cells, our bodies are not as efficient as they once were in producing them, and our organs suffer.

Apoptosis
A form of cell death in which a predictable sequence of events leads to the eradication of cells without the release of harmful substances into the surrounding tissues.

In 1994, researchers in Sydney, Australia, treated human cells with carnosine to test its effect on growth, shape, and life span. They found that cells grown in a carnosine-rich environment maintained their "youthful appearance." Although the Hayflick limit still applied, cells lived longer between divisions. The researchers also noted that carnosine could rejuvenate old cells, and when these were later removed from the carnosine solution they became aged once again.

Carnosine Prevents Strokes

Strokes are the third leading cause of death among Americans. About half a million people suffer strokes annually, and more than 165,000 of them are fatal. Most of these cases—about 80 percent—are what is known as ischemic strokes, meaning they are caused by an interruption in the flow of blood to the brain. In most cases, blood flow is blocked by a clot, so in a sense, an ischemic stroke is like a heart attack in the brain.

There are three arteries that supply the brain

with blood—carotid, vertebral, and basilar. Like the arteries in the heart, the brain's arteries can also become filled with plaque. The site where the plaque settles in the artery becomes narrowed, and a clot may form there. Or the clot may come from another part of the body and eventually lodge near the brain. In either case, the result is the same. Brain cell and brain tissue are deprived of oxygen and die. Two factors— the extent of the brain damage and where it occurs in the brain—determine whether the individual will resume normal functions, require assistance for ordinary activities, or need permanent hospitalization. Unfortunately, only a small minority—about 10 percent—of all stroke victims fall into the first category, and make a full recovery. Roughly 50 percent can return home, but need help with day-to-day tasks, while the remaining 40 percent require such extensive assistance that they must live in an institution.

The symptoms of stroke run the gamut. Some people experience transient ischemic strokes (TIA) prior to a more serious episode. TIAs are caused by a temporary interference in blood flow to the brain, but share several stroke symptoms. Weakness or paralysis in an arm or leg, loss of coordination, numbness, dizziness, loss of balance, or disrupted vision in one or both eyes are typical signs of a TIA. These symptoms should be taken seriously and a doctor should evaluate the individual as soon as possible.

When a full-blown stroke occurs, an individual may experience these symptoms, as well as a sudden, exceedingly painful headache, an inability to speak or understand what is being said to them, or weakness on one side of the body. There are many options when it comes to avoiding stroke, and carnosine is one of them.

The Russian journal *Biochemistry* devoted much of a recent issue to carnosine. In one review summarizing previous research, the authors concluded that carnosine has "pronounced anti-ischemic effects" in the brain and heart, thanks to its antioxidant and membrane-protecting abilities. They noted that in animal studies involving experimentally induced strokes, carnosine decreased the number of deaths and protected brain cells from oxygen-deprivation damage.

Ischemia
Inadequate blood supply (circulation) to a specific area caused by blockage of the blood vessels.

More recently, a new study from Israel investigated the effectiveness of carnosine, and a related substance known as homocarnosine, on ischemic events *in* human cells. Both compounds provided significant protection, sparing 50 percent of the damage that typically occurs when these cells are deprived of oxygen.

Acute kidney failure due to medication, internal bleeding, or dehydration can cause a sort of ischemic reaction in the kidneys, with too little blood flow and sudden loss of kidney function. When acute kidney failure occurs, an individual may feel fatigued or drowsy, may feel nauseous, and may produce very little urine. A recent study from Japan found that pretreating animals with carnosine prior to cutting off the blood supply to one kidney provided considerable protection. Kidneys of the carnosine-treated animals resumed normal functioning more quickly, and damage to the organ was minimized, with higher doses of carnosine providing greater protection.

Carnosine Protects against Cataracts

As we age, the lens covering our eyes becomes less flexible, thicker, and, as a result, less transparent. The loss of transparency means the retina receives less light or only distorted light rays, causing a gradual loss of vision.

Not surprisingly, the process of cataract development involves proteins gone wrong. In fact, units of protein form clusters, and these, combined with the lens's reduced flexibility, make the eye appear to be covered by a cloudy film. Cataracts are commonly removed surgically, but several studies show that carnosine eyedrops can treat and even prevent cataract formation.

In a study reported in *Drug Research and Development*, forty-nine individuals with cataracts were divided into two groups. One was given eyedrops containing a form of carnosine (N-acetylcarnosine) twice daily, while the control group was given placebo eyedrops that looked like the real thing but contained no carnosine. After six months, an impressive 90 percent of the carnosine-treated eyes had improved vision, and glare sensitivity was reduced, sometimes by as much as 100 percent! In the control group, which received no treatment, there was significant deterioration of vision. Researchers also noted that the carnosine eyedrops were well tolerated by nearly all the patients.

There is still a great deal about the aging process that is not clear, but scientists are working hard to develop anti-aging strategies. Based on what is currently known about carnosine, it should play a major role in preventing much of the damage that occurs in the body as we grow older. But carnosine can benefit young, healthy individuals in a number of ways, as we will see in the next chapter.

CHAPTER 6

CARNOSINE FOR OVERALL GOOD HEALTH

With nearly 1,000 studies on carnosine, it should not be surprising to learn that it benefits a wide range of functions in the body. Although it has been widely used by athletes and bodybuilders because of its outstanding ability to prevent muscle fatigue, and therefore make work-outs more effective, carnosine is creating a stir among advocates of anti-aging medicine, too. In part, this is due to its antioxidant effects, as well as to carnosine's ability to prevent protein-damaging glycation, two processes involved in aging.

You don't have to be a bodybuilder, a senior citizen, or even middle-aged, to benefit from carnosine, though. Although they tend to be more common among the elderly, heart disease, cancer, ulcers, and inflammation can affect the young and old alike. In all these cases, carnosine has been shown to be effective. Let's take a closer look at some of the science behind these claims.

Our Most Common Concern: Cardiovascular Disease

The human cardiovascular system consists of the heart, which is essentially two pumps, and a series of blood vessels of varying sizes. We have about 60,000 miles of blood vessels in our bodies, including the arteries, veins, and capillaries. Oxygen-rich blood moves away from the heart through the arteries, delivers oxygen to cells throughout the body, and then returns to the heart via the veins. A normal, healthy human heart beats an astonishing 100,000 times each day, circulating the 6.5 pints of blood in the human body.

Both chambers of the heart—known as the atrium and ventricle—are muscles. Arteries, veins, and capillaries are all essentially tubes, designed to do specific jobs. Because the arteries have to bear the brunt of blood being forced out of the heart during contractions, they are sturdy, strong vessels. Our veins have thinner walls, and the capillary walls are actually quite delicate so that oxygen and various chemicals can flow out and be delivered to the cells.

When all is working well, the cardiovascular system is an amazingly efficient and powerful machine. Exercise is one key to a healthy heart. Because it is a muscle, your heart is strengthened by aerobic exercise. But a sedentary lifestyle, poor diet, stress, and aging all take a toll on the heart, making it vulnerable to problems in several areas.

Atherosclerosis, or hardening of the arteries, is one of most common causes of cardiovascular disease. According to the Centers for Disease Control and Prevention (CDC), cardiovascular disease kills more Americans than any other illness, with some 700,000 fatalities in a typical year. Although the arteries are built to be both tough and flexible, they can become compromised by deposits of plaque. These are small clumps that form when cholesterol, a waxy form of fat, combines with other substances. As plaque accumulates, arteries become narrower, just like a clogged drain in the sink.

Plaque
A semihardened accumulation of substances from fluids that circulate through an area, such as a blood vessel.

To make matters worse, inflammation can complicate matters by increasing the amount of C-reactive protein (CRP) in the body. This unstable substance contributes to the clots that can lodge in a narrowed artery. Eventually, the artery may become so blocked that blood flow is limited, or even prevented altogether, causing a heart attack.

How Carnosine Can Help the Heart

Three separate studies illustrate a variety of ways that carnosine can keep our hearts healthy. Let's start by repeating two important facts—one, the heart is a muscle, and two, carnosine is found in high concentrations in muscle tissue, especially in the heart. This is not a coincidence, say experts, but nature's way of protecting this vitally essential organ. Unfortunately, the aging process causes carnosine levels to drop, causing many of the complications we take for granted as part of growing older. The good news is that carnosine has been proven to protect against a number of these occurrences.

The first study, which was published in the journal *Nutrition*, found that carnosine relaxed arteries that had been chemically constricted for the experiment. This is an important benefit, because blood flows more normally in relaxed arteries than those that are tight and narrow.

Secondly, researchers at Wake Forest University School of Medicine examined the effects of carnosine on the heart's ability to contract effectively, a primary factor in patients with ischemic heart disease and inflammatory conditions such as sepsis. The problem behind inadequate heart contractions has to do with faulty monitoring of calcium levels in the cells. The researchers found that carnosine not only improved contractions in the heart muscle but also stabilized the calcium response in heart cells.

In the third clinical trial, Italian researchers discovered that carnosine's antioxidant abilities could protect LDL cholesterol from a specific form of free-radical damage. Although LDL (low-density lipoprotein) cholesterol is usually considered "bad," it is not inherently unhealthy and actually serves important functions in the body. LDL cholesterol becomes a problem only after it is oxidized by free radicals, making it more likely to form artery-clogging plaque. Carnosine, as the researchers noted, helped minimize this process, even at levels no higher than those typically found in our bodies.

Conquering Cancer with Carnosine

Although it is a complex disease that can affect almost any organ in the body, cancer begins as a single cell. Instead of behaving normally, however, a cancer cell multiplies, creating a tumor. Eventually, the tumor can be responsible for cancer spreading throughout the body. Our knowledge of cancer today could fill volumes, but a cure remains elusive. Because of that, experts say that prevention should be our number one priority. The best place to begin is with two elements of lifestyle—diet and smoking. Some 35 percent of all cancer deaths each year are related to poor diet, while another 30 percent are linked to tobacco, so by simply cleaning up our dietary act and giving up tobacco, more than half of all cancers could be eliminated.

Cancer
Abnormal growth of cells, which tend to reproduce in an uncontrolled manner and, in some cases, to spread (metastasize).

The exact role of diet is still open to some debate, but a growing body of research shows that people who consume the most antioxidant-rich fruits and vegetables are less likely to develop cancer. Experts believe that one reason fruits and vegetables minimize cancer risk is because they are rich in antioxidants. Clearly, antioxidant supplements should provide protection, too, and a recent study in the journal *Nutrition and Cancer* supports this theory. Researchers at University of North Carolina, Chapel Hill, found that breast cancer patients who took supplements of vitamins C and E for more than three years had a reduced risk both of the disease reappearing and of dying from it.

Of course, as we have seen, carnosine is an extraordinary antioxidant. And recent studies show that it does provide protection against cancer at the cellular level. One of these, published recently in *Cancer Letters*, found that carnosine prevented two types of free-radical cell damage that has been linked to both cancer and neurodegenerative diseases, such as Parkinson's and Alzheimer's.

The diet-cancer connection is especially relevant to carnosine. As we have seen, several types of meat are rich in the substance, but many people are reducing their meat intake or eliminating it from their diet altogether. Although the findings remain controversial, meat consumption has been linked to several types of cancer. In addition, some people want to avoid the hormones and antibiotics found in a great deal of meat today. Carnosine supplements can make up for a lack of meat in the diet.

Ulcers and Carnosine

About 4 million Americans live with peptic ulcers, which are essentially open sores affecting the lining of the stomach. A second type, occurring in the first portion of the small intestine, or duodenum, are called duodenal ulcers. The symptoms of peptic ulcers vary, but usually involve heartburn, nausea, vomiting, and/or a bloated feeling. Duodenal ulcers can cause pain in the back, as well as nausea and vomiting.

Ulcers are not particularly dangerous, in and of themselves, although they can become perforated and create a medical emergency. But they definitely cause discomfort. Worse, ulcers and the antacids many people take to ease their pain disrupt digestion and interfere with proper absorption of nutrients.

Until 1994, ulcers were believed to be caused by an unfortunate combination of stress and stomach acid. Antacids were prescribed, and were often taken for years with little improvement. Now we know that nearly all ulcers are actually due to inflammation of the stomach lining caused by the *Helicobacter pylori* (*H. pylori*) bacterium. There are three different methods of eradicating *H. pylori*, and all involve taking antibiotics and other drugs for about two weeks.

H. pylori
A bacterium that is the cause of about 80 percent of stomach ulcers and nearly all duodenal ulcers.

Several animal studies have shown that a combination of carnosine and the mineral zinc not only promotes healing of existing ulcers but also provides protection against their development. Furthermore, a human clinical trial involving sixty patients with *H. pylori* infections compared the results of the standard antibiotic treatment alone and with the addition of carnosine and zinc. After one week, the carnosine-zinc group experienced a 94 percent rate of improvement, versus a 74 percent rate in the antibiotics-only group.

Promoting Immunity

The world we live in is filled with a wide variety of microorganisms, such as bacteria and viruses. Some of these are beneficial, but others can be life threatening. To protect us, nature has provided a powerful shield in the immune system, which attacks and conquers many of the substances we encounter.

Our immune systems extend throughout the body, in a network of lymph glands and other vessels in the front and back of the neck, groin, and inside certain organs. Bone marrow, the spleen, and the thymus gland all produce infection-battling white blood cells that roam throughout this system, looking for trouble spots.

When the immune system is functioning at its peak, it is remarkably effective. But there are a number of factors that can diminish its effectiveness, including stress, a poor diet, lack of rest, certain medications, and aging.

Immune System

A complex system that works to identify, find, and kill invaders, ranging from infections to foreign substances.

Carnosine can help support the immune system, according to two Japanese studies. In one, animals' immune systems were weakened by many of the same things that can affect humans, including chemotherapy drugs, yet carnosine enhanced the subjects' immunity. In the second trial, older animals with naturally weakened immune systems also got boosts in immunity from carnosine.

Carnosine Combats Stress

Stress is especially hard on the immune system. Certain aspects of the immune system, such as natural killer (NK) cells, function less effectively when we experience stress. Stress can result from unfortunate or negative events—such as job loss, divorce, or death of a loved one—as well as happy occurrences, such as getting married, moving, or starting a new job.

While a small amount of stress can be energizing, modern life is filled with a seemingly endless number of events that can leave us feeling "stressed out." Inside the body, stress causes the adrenal glands to work overtime, producing several hormones, including epinephrine, norepinephrine, and cortisol. Epinephrine increases the heart rate, blood pressure, and blood glucose levels in preparation for "fight or flight." Similarly, norepinephrine also boosts blood pressure, while cortisol can alter the way we process carbohydrates, proteins, and fats, leading some experts to conclude that it is linked to weight gain and to the difficulty people have with losing weight.

Earlier research into carnosine's effects on stress found two ways it is beneficial. One study from Japan determined that animals treated with carnosine and then subjected to a stressful event still produced cortisol in response, but it was metabolized and removed from their bodies more quickly than in untreated animals. A second study, conducted in Russia, found that carnosine protected against the free-radical oxidation of fats in the body during stressful periods.

Furthermore, a recent study noted that carnosine decreased blood pressure in animals bred to have high blood pressure. As a result, the researchers speculated that carnosine's prevalence in muscles may be nature's way of moderating blood pressure. While this study needs to be repeated and confirmed in humans, it presents a promising possibility for new blood pressure treatments that can reduce the effects of stress.

CHAPTER 7

CARNOSINE: TREATING THE UNTREATABLE

Although health experts don't always see eye to eye, there are two areas where you are likely to find little argument. One is the fact that the graying of America as the baby boomers head for senior citizen status is virtually guaranteed to create a health-care crisis. Millions of people will reach old age at a time when life expectancies are longer than ever. At the same time, cures or effective treatments for many of the most common chronic conditions are elusive. Consider, for example, that between 1990 and 2030, the number of people over the age of sixty will soar by about 75 percent in the industrialized world. Since it is well established that the likelihood of developing Alzheimer's disease increases as we grow older, the number of people diagnosed with the disease, now at 4.5 million, is expected to rise along with our aging population. The same is true of other conditions associated with advanced years, such as Parkinson's disease. Understandably, this is of great concern to health-care authorities.

At the other end of the age spectrum, there is another issue brewing that experts agree is at crisis proportions, and that is autism. An incapacitating developmental brain disorder, autism has gone from being a rare diagnosis to the number-one disability among children in several states. In California, for example, the number of autism cases is doubling every four years, with no end in sight. In Ohio, there was an increase of nearly 14,000 percent between the years 1992 and 2002, while the rate in Illinois soared by an astonishing 76,040 percent in the same time period!

The symptoms of autism vary widely, but often include some degree of withdrawal from others, and difficulties with learning, language, and/or social behavior. Although childhood vaccines have been suggested as a possible cause, no one can say definitively where autism comes from, and there is no cure.

At first glance, it may seem that Alzheimer's, Parkinson's, and autism have nothing in common. But they actually do share one thing: carnosine is showing great promise as a treatment for all three.

Avoiding Alzheimer's with Carnosine

Alzheimer's disease is a dreaded condition affecting some 4 million Americans, most of them elderly. Alzheimer's is actually the most common form of a condition known as dementia, a progressive, degenerative disease of the brain that is considered irreversible. Although science is learning more about the condition each year, many questions remain and there is little in the way of treatment options.

Early-Onset Alzheimer's Disease
The term used for Alzheimer's disease that occurs in people in their forties and fifties. About 10 percent of Alzheimer's patients are in this category.

Alzheimer's is characterized by memory loss, personality changes, and impaired mental functions. This is believed to be due to several factors, including the death of brain cells, insufficient supplies of the neurotransmitter acetylcholine, and an accumulation of plaque consisting of clusters of dead neurons filled with the protein beta-amyloid.

Carnosine is showing great promise at treating Alzheimer's because of its ability to prevent protein glycation and the formation of advanced glycation end products (AGEs). For example, researchers in Germany found that AGE-inhibitors, including carnosine, could prevent beta-amyloid clusters. And they noted that in clinical trials with Alzheimer's patients, those taking AGE-inhibitors reported improved memory and mental functions.

Preventing Parkinson's Disease with Carnosine

Parkinson's disease is quite common among those over age sixty, occurring in one out of every 200 people. A neurodegenerative disease, Parkinson's disease involves a loss of brain cells in an area of the brain where a number of essential neurotransmitters are produced. It is characterized by slight tremors, usually in the hands, and fatigue, both of which can worsen over time. As we saw in Chapter 3, a 34-year-long study of more than 8,000 men and women found a link between Parkinson's disease and high consumption of fruit and fruit drinks. As yet, researchers do not know why this link exists. The team that conducted the study believes it may have to do with pesticides and herbicides found on fruit; other experts point to the large quantities of fructose and high-fructose corn syrup (HFCS) found in many fruit beverages (as well as many other foods). Both fructose and HFCS cause protein damage and development of free-radical producing AGEs.

Parkinson's Disease

A slowly progressive neurologic disease characterized by tremors, awkward gait and posture, muscle weakness, and low production of the neurotransmitter dopamine.

While experts work to clarify the link between fruit and Parkinson's disease, advances are being made on the carnosine front. Some researchers believe that free-radical damage is responsible for the death of brain cells that occurs in Parkinson's. A new study from Korea shows that antioxidants, including carnosine, inhibit protein damage, leading the research team to conclude that these compounds merit further exploration as treatments for Parkinson's. And scientists at Florida State University determined that carnosine has the ability to manage zinc and copper, two essential minerals that can contribute to Alzheimer's, Parkinson's, stroke, and seizures if levels are not kept in check.

Carnosine for Autism

So far, there has been only one study showing that carnosine improved symptoms of autism, but the results occurred quickly and were impressive. At the end of the eight-week study, there was a nearly 30 percent increase in social interaction, and a 16 percent improvement in behavior, language, and communication in the group taking carnosine. Although this study involved only thirty-one children, the pediatric neurologist who led the research, Michael Chez, says he has used carnosine on about 1,000 autistic children and reports a 90 percent success rate. Epilepsy, brain injury, and central processing disorders also respond to treatment with carnosine, says Chez.

Clearly, it is not an accident that some of the highest levels of carnosine are found in the brain. As scientists continue to unravel its mysteries, we should gain a better understanding of carnosine's role in brain health. In the meantime, carnosine supplements can provide protection without side effects, as we will see in the next chapter.

CHAPTER 8

CHOOSING CARNOSINE SUPPLEMENTS

Before looking at dosage details, let's review carnosine's benefits to determine who should take it and why. In general, within our bodies, carnosine is most abundant in the brain, eyes, and muscles, including the heart. Since carnosine levels drop significantly as we age, it makes sense to take supplements as a means of providing continued protection. And since the only dietary source of carnosine is meat, vegetarians are especially likely to have low levels of this nutrient.

In addition, there are several specific reasons to consider carnosine supplements. As we have seen, carnosine is a powerful antioxidant, with an ability to quench free radicals as well as protect cell membranes against free-radical damage. This attribute alone makes it a fine addition to any daily supplement regimen, since we are all faced with exposure to dangerous free radicals.

Because of its antioxidant abilities, carnosine is also a valuable nutrient for anyone suffering from conditions related to inflammation. These include heart disease, arthritis, diabetes, allergies, Alzheimer's, obesity, asthma, ulcers, and certain cancers. Because inflammation produces free radicals, people with chronic inflammatory conditions require more antioxidant protection than individuals without these ailments.

In addition to fighting free radicals, carnosine has a dramatic effect on the protein-damaging process known as glycation. Essentially, glycation contributes to the complications associated with aging by damaging proteins and DNA and preventing them from functioning properly. Although it is as invisible as the havoc wreaked by free radicals, glycation affects the entire body, causing, among other things, damage to blood vessels, Alzheimer's-related damage in the brain, stiffening in joint cartilage, and reduced collagen in the skin, which allows wrinkles to form. Carnosine has been shown to inhibit glycation in a number of experiments. Even if it was not a powerhouse antioxidant, this fact alone makes carnosine a vitally important supplement for anyone who wants to age well and remain in good health for as long as possible.

Another area where carnosine shines is its positive effect on muscles. Although it has long been popular with sports enthusiasts and bodybuilders, there is no reason why elite athletes should be the only ones enjoying carnosine's benefits. Carnosine does not add bulk to muscles; it simply enables them to work longer and harder. This is important for two reasons. One, people who have difficulty with weight management can benefit from exercise and stronger muscles, which burn more calories than fat. Two, in older people, the muscle-wasting condition known as sarcopenia is shaping up as a major factor in debilitating falls—and related broken bones—among the elderly. The best way to avoid sarcopenia is by keeping muscles strong throughout life, and carnosine can help.

Muscular Dystrophy
One of several genetic diseases distinguished by progressive weakness and deterioration of the muscles that control movement.

Although research is in its preliminary stages, carnosine's special affinity for muscle has been shown to strengthen animals with neuromuscular disorders, such as forms of muscular dystrophy and Parkinson's disease. It is possible that one day carnosine—alone or combined with other substances—may make these devastating disorders a thing of the past.

Finally, the promising results of a study showing children with autism benefit from carnosine may lead to a solution for this increasingly common condition.

Determining Dosage

Because carnosine is a relatively new supplement in this country, there are no firm guidelines regarding dosage. Keep in mind, however, that carnosine has been extensively studied. Side effects are rare, usually involving a slight shakiness in muscles, and these have only been reported at high doses. The only condition attributed to an overload of carnosine, carnosinemia, is in - herited and cannot be caused by taking carnosine supplements. At this time, there are no known drug interactions involving carnosine.

Carnosinemia
A rare genetic condition characterized by an accumulation of carnosine in the body.

If you are currently in good health, 150 to 200 milligrams (mg) of carnosine daily should provide adequate protection against everyday free radicals and glycation. Will you see dramatic changes? It's hard to say. Just as oxidation and glycation quietly occur behind the scenes, so too does carnosine work to minimize damage without much fanfare. (By the way, although carnosine can be obtained from meat, supplements are available in synthetic form, so vegetarians and vegans can take advantage of this nutrient.)

Higher doses of carnosine—500 milligrams to

1,500 milligrams, for example—are sometimes recommended, but several experts suggest staying with lower amounts. And one small clinical trial found that doses greater than 500 milligrams were actually less effective than the 100- to 200-milligram standard amount. Of course, anyone who is currently taking medication and/or being treated by a physician should discuss adding specific supplements beforehand. Unfortunately, many doctors are not aware of carnosine, and may need to review the literature before making a recommendation.

Finally, the carnosine dosage in the study on autism was 400 milligrams given twice daily, along with 50 international units (IU) of vitamin E and 5 milligrams of zinc. Although carnosine is a naturally occurring substance, it has not been widely researched in children and its long-term effects as a supplement are unknown, so it makes sense to discuss these issues thoroughly with a physician before treating a child.

Complementing Carnosine

One consideration to keep in mind is that carnosine interacts well with other antioxidants, such as vitamin A or beta-carotene, vitamins C and E, selenium, zinc, and others. Taking a variety of antioxidants increases their effectiveness, and helps minimize the overwhelming numbers of free radicals our bodies must deal with every day.

Less Heat, Less Aging

You can make carnosine even more effective by making a few dietary changes. In Chapter 3, we saw how damaging sugar, and especially high fructose corn syrup (HFCS), can be to health, because it increases glycation. Passing up packaged and processed foods, with their abundant amounts of HFCS, is an excellent way to minimize glycation. Also, sodas are not healthy choices for a number of reasons, but the dark-colored ones have an added downside: they are likely to contain caramelized flavorings filled with glycation's free-radical producing byproducts, AGEs.

You can also reduce glycation and consumption of AGEs by avoiding foods, especially meat, cooked at high temperatures. According to a recent report published in the prestigious *Proceedings of the National Academy of Sciences,* foods cooked at high temperatures contain more AGEs than those cooked at lower temperatures, and consuming these foods on a regular basis could result in low-grade, chronic inflammation in the body.

Grilling, which involves very high temperatures, should be replaced by boiling, steaming, or sautéing, and meat should be sliced thinly to further reduce AGEs. Time is also a factor in the development of AGEs. The faster meat is cooked, the fewer of these toxins are created, which means the traditional holiday turkey that roasts for hours in the oven is not very healthy fare.

CONCLUSION

This book may be your first introduction to carnosine. If so, congratulations for seeking out cutting-edge health information. With carnosine's many benefits, as well as the promise it is showing in treating difficult conditions, it's hard to believe that it has taken more than 100 years for this nutrient to become an overnight success!

Whether you want to live to be 100—or more—or simply want to live as well as possible for as long as possible, carnosine can help. The simple fact that carnosine is most heavily concentrated in the brain, eyes, heart, and skeletal muscle suggests that it is nature's way of protecting these vitally important parts of the body. Maintaining adequate levels of carnosine is a smart way to support nature's plan.

Don't be surprised to see carnosine getting more attention from the media in the years ahead. Studies are ongoing, and there will very likely be new developments on the carnosine front soon. Meanwhile, there is abundant research showing that a little carnosine can go a long way toward enhancing our overall health and improving symptoms of some serious health concerns. All in all, carnosine is clearly a supplement whose time has come.

SELECTED
REFERENCES

Aldini G., P. Granata, and M. Carini. "Detoxification of cytotoxic alpha, beta-unsaturated aldehydes by carnosine: Characterization of conjugated adducts by electrospray ionization tandem mass spectrometry and detection by liquid chromatography/mass spectrometry in rat skeletal muscle." *Journal of Mass Spectrometry* 2002 Dec; 37(12):1219–1228.

Boldyrev, A.A., S.C. Gallant, and G.T. Sukhich. "Carnosine, the protective, anti-aging peptide." *Bioscience Reports* 1999 Dec; 19(6):581–587.

Chez, M.G., C. P. Buchanan, M. C. Aimonovitch, et al. "Double-blind, placebo-controlled study of L-carnosine supplementation in children with autistic spectrum disorders." *Journal of Child Neurology* 2002 Nov; 17(11):833–837.

Davison, K. K., E. S. Ford, M. E. Cogswell, et al. "Percentage of body fat and body mass index are associated with mobility limitations in people aged 70 and older from NHANES II." *Journal of the American Geriatric Society* 2002 Nov; 50(11):1802–1809.

Elliott, S.S., N.L. Keim, J.S. Stern, et al. "Fructose, weight gain, and the insulin resistance syndrome." *American Journal of Clinical Nutrition* 2002 Nov; 76(5):911–922.

Gallant, S., M. Semyonova, and M. Yuneva. "Carnosine as a potential anti-senescence drug." *Biochemistry* (Mosc) 2000 Jul; 65(7):866–868.

Gille, J. J., P. Pasman, C. G. van Berkel, et al. "Effect of antioxidants on hyperoxia-induced chromosomal breakage in Chinese hamster ovary cells: Protection by carnosine." *Mutagenesis* 1991 Jul; 6(4):313–318.

Hipkiss, A.R., C. Brownson, M.F. Bertani, et al. "Reaction of carnosine with aged proteins: another protective process." *Annals of the New York Academy of Science* 2002 Apr; 959:285–294.

Holliday, R. and G.A. McFarland. "A role for carnosine in cellular maintenance." *Biochemistry* (Mosc) 2000 Jul; 65(7):843–848.

Kang, J.H., and K.S. Kim. "Enhanced oligomerization of the alpha-synuclein mutant by the Cu, Zn-superoxide dismutase and hydrogen peroxide system." *Molecular Cell* 2003 Feb 28; 15(1):87–93.

Marchis, S.D., C. Modena, P. Peretto, et al. "Carnosine-related dipeptides in neurons and glia." *Biochemistry* (Mosc) 2000 Jul; 65(7):824–833.

McFarland, G.A. and R. Holliday. "Retardation of the senescence of cultured human diploid fibroblasts by carnosine." *Experimental Cell Research* 1994 Jun; 212(2):167-175.

Seidler, N.W., and G.S. Yeargans. "Effects of thermal denaturation on protein glycation." *Life Sciences* 2002 Mar 1; 70(15):1789–1799.

Shulman, J.M., L.M. Shulman, W.J. Weiner, et al. "From fruit fly to bedside: Translating lessons from Drosophila models of neurodegenerative disease." *Current Opinions in Neurology* 2003 Aug; 16(4): 443–449.

Stuerenburg, H.J. "The roles of carnosine in aging of skeletal muscle and in neuromuscular diseases." *Biochemistry* (Mosc) 2000 Jul; 65(7):862–865.

Suzuki, Y., O. Ito, N. Mukai, et al. "High level of skeletal muscle carnosine contributes to the latter half of exercise performance during 30-s maximal cycle ergometer sprinting." *Japanese Journal of Physiology* 2002 Apr; 52(2):199–205.

Trombley, P.Q., M.S. Horning, and L.J. Blakemore. "Interactions between carnosine and zinc and copper: Implications for neuromodulation and neuroprotection." *Biochemistry* (Mosc) 2000 Jul;65(7): 807–816.

Wang, A.M., C. Ma, Z.H. Xie, et al. "Use of carnosine as a natural anti-senescence drug for human beings." *Biochemistry* (Mosc) 2000 Jul; 65(7):869–871.

Yeargans, G.S. and N.W. Seidler. "Carnosine promotes the heat denaturation of glycated protein." *Biochemical and Biophysical Research Communications* 2003 Jan 3; 300(1):75–80.

Yuneva, A.O., G.G. Kramarenko, T.V. Vetreshchak, et al. "Effect of carnosine on Drosophila melanogaster lifespan." *Bulletin of Experimental Biology and Medicine* 2002 Jun; 133(6):559–561.

OTHER BOOKS
AND RESOURCES

Braverman, Eric. *The Healing Nutrients Within: Your Guide to the Best-Stocked Drugstore of All— The Human Body.* North Bergen, N.J.: Basic Health, 2002.

Challem, Jack. *The Inflammation Syndrome: The Complete Nutritional Program to Prevent and Reverse Heart Disease, Arthritis, Diabetes, Allergies, and, Asthma.* New York: Wiley, 2003.

Challem, Jack, Berkson, Burton, and Smith, Melissa Diane. *Syndrome X: The Complete Nutritional Program to Prevent and Reverse Insulin Resistance.* New York: Wiley, 2000.

GreatLife Magazine
Consumer magazine with articles on vitamins, minerals, herbs, and foods.
Available for free at many health and natural food stores.

Let's Live Magazine
Consumer magazine with emphasis on the health benefits of vitamins, minerals, and herbs.

Customer service:
1-800-676-4333
P.O. Box 74908
Los Angeles, CA 90004
Subscriptions: 12 issues per year, $19.95 in the U.S.; $31.95 outside the U.S.

Physical Magazine

Magazine oriented to bodybuilders and other serious athletes.

Customer service:

1-800-676-4333

P.O. Box 74908

Los Angeles, CA 90004

Subscriptions: 12 issues per year, $19.95 in the U.S.; $31.95 outside the U.S.

The Nutrition Reporter™ newsletter

Monthly newsletter that summarizes recent medical research on vitamins, minerals, and herbs.

Customer service:

P.O. Box 30246

Tucson, AZ 85751-0246

e-mail: jack@thenutritionreporter.com

www.nutritionreporter.com

Subscriptions: 12 issues per year, $26 in the U.S.; $32 U.S. or $48 CNC for Canada; $38 for other countries.

For more information on sarcopenia, go to:
www.sarcopenia.com.

For more information on health and fitness, contact:

The American Heart Association

7272 Greenville Avenue

Dallas, TX 75231

800-242-8721

www.americanheart.org *or* www.justmove.org.

INDEX

Printed in the USA
CPSIA information can be obtained
at www.ICGtesting.com
JSHW051957150824
68134JS00050B/77